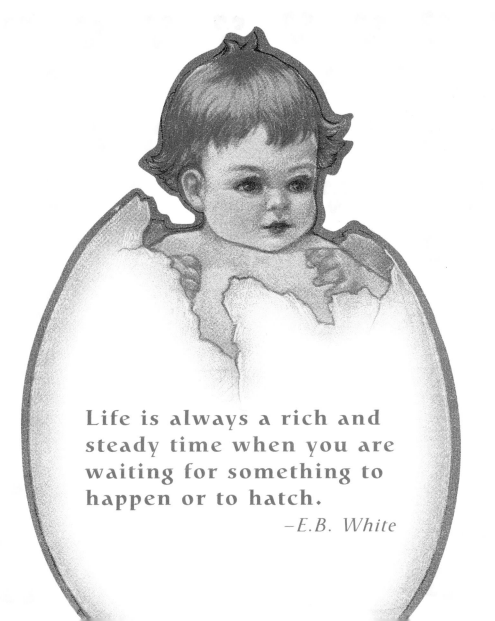

Life is always a rich and steady time when you are waiting for something to happen or to hatch.

—E.B. White

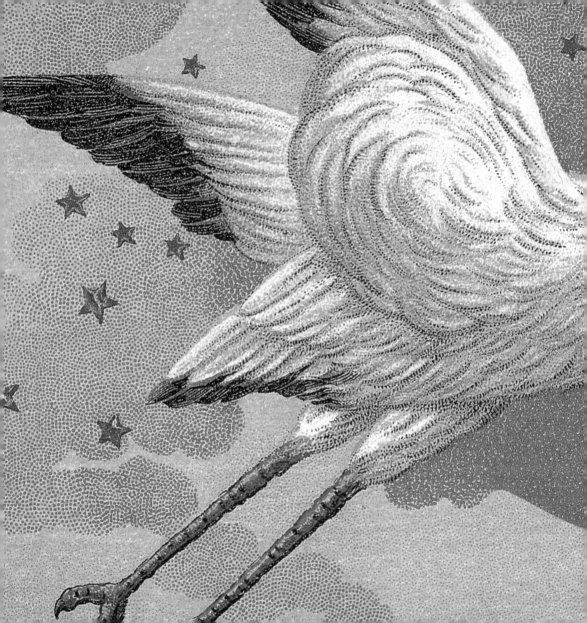

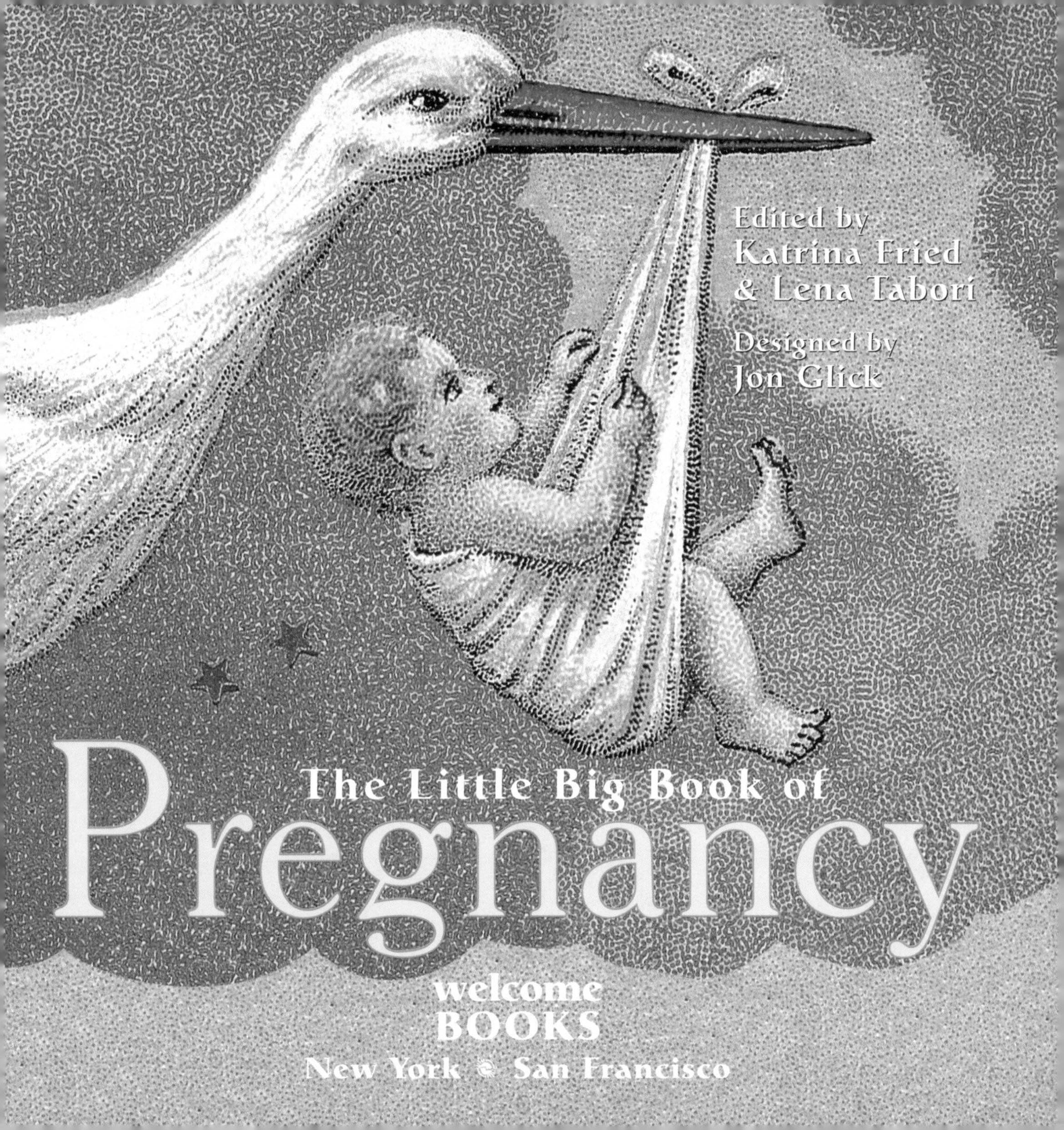

Edited by
Katrina Fried
& Lena Tabori

Designed by
Jon Glick

The Little Big Book of
Pregnancy

welcome
BOOKS
New York ● San Francisco

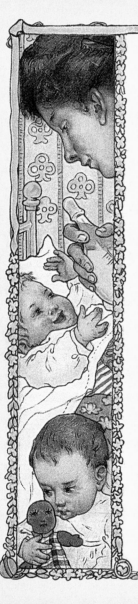

CONTENTS

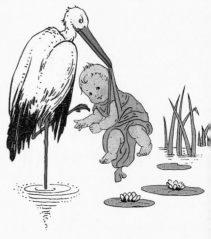

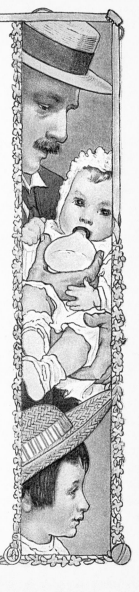

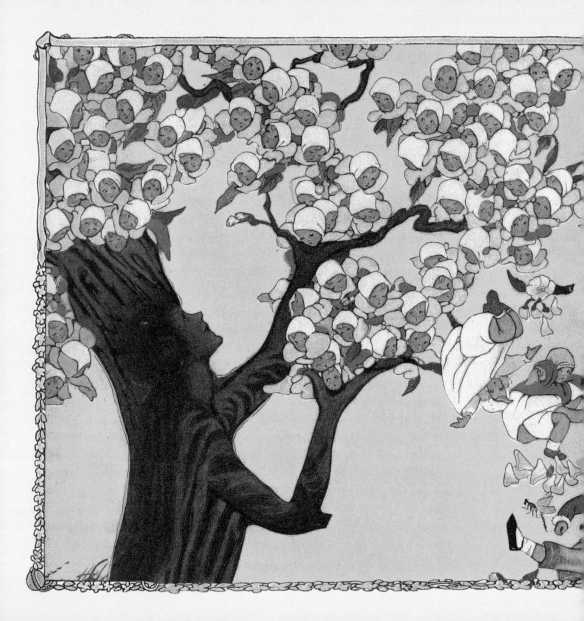

ACTIVITIES

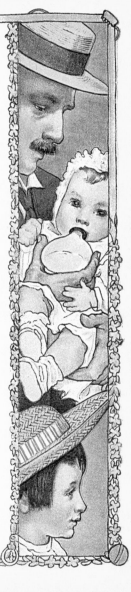

RECIPES

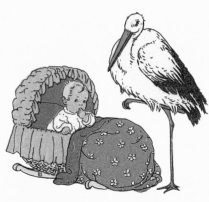

CAN YOU THINK OF ANY REASON why my boss—who also happens to be my mother—would assign me to co-edit *The Little Big Book of Pregnancy*? Well, I have an idea or two. I am twenty-nine years old and just celebrated my sixth wedding anniversary. My husband and I have recently purchased our first home and...we don't have any children yet. Let's see...what possible motive could she have?

Well, I'll tell you a secret if you promise not to tell my mom: I'm ready to start a family. The truth is, researching and editing this book *did* help me set aside any lingering doubts I may have harbored about becoming a mother. The more I read, the more I began

Looking Forward

to fantasize about all the "firsts" that come with pregnancy: feeling the baby kick, choosing a name, big breasts, growing huge and hormonal, shopping for two, eating for two, giving birth, breast-feeding, and finally, seeing my husband hold our baby in his arms. Could it really get any better than that?

It might seem unusual for a woman who has yet to experience pregnancy to edit a compilation on the subject, but actually it makes great sense. I approached this assignment armed with years' worth of my own questions about becoming a mother. I poured through the recollections, stories, and advice of amazing women; I made lists of the most useful and enjoyable activities and information; I asked for suggestions on every subject from all the moms and moms-to-be I know; and then I selected and commissioned the material I would want to read, learn, and benefit from during my own pregnancy. The result is a beautifully designed volume that celebrates every aspect of those enchanted nine months—the exciting, the frightening, the spiritual, and the physical.

Filled with interesting traditions, entertaining old wives' tales, fresh advice, original recipes, and the most inspiring literary excerpts, stories, and essays, *The Little Big Book of Pregnancy* is as much for the woman about to experience her first pregnancy as it is for the mom having child number three. It is also my mother's gift to me, and just maybe it will result in a very special gift to my mother....

Katrina Fried
the daughter

FIRST I WAS EXHAUSTED, sleeping the moment I came home from work. Then I was irritable; there was nothing my poor husband could do that was right. When my breasts started to become larger—I had been waiting most of my life for that—I knew I was pregnant. I didn't feel so well, but at least I had the breasts—delicious, unexpected, and entirely welcome.

By the time three months had passed, my waistline had begun to go, but I felt fantastic. I was an Amazon. I was glorious. I could conquer anything…until my ninth month rolled around. I had become heavy and impatient. Thank God for Lamaze class: dozens of women maneuvering through the revolving doors of that old hotel on 42nd street, winding their way to the ancient and wise Elizabeth Bing, who waited patiently while we took deep breaths and our husbands massaged our backs and taught us when and how to pant.

I miscalculated all my contractions when I went into labor with my first daughter and was nine centimeters dilated by the time I reached the hospital. As I was wheeled into the delivery room I turned to my husband and said, "Did you hear that lion roar?" "That was no lion," he said, "that was you." She was rosy and pink. She looked like a little Russian peasant. Definitely Natasha. Two years later, back in the hospital I'd scarcely experienced the first time, I waited for my second little one. And wait I did, all through the night, watching the tugboats and the lights on the East River, falling asleep between contractions. By 8:10 A.M. that Saturday morning Katrina was in my arms.

Then and now, the truth is the same: I loved my pregnancies and I didn't want to miss a minute of my births. I was lucky to be able to have my children naturally. I wanted to breastfeed them and I did, pumping out milk when I went back to work. The memory of the rocking chair with them nuzzling and touching my face with their little hands…it's the best thing. Just the best thing.

Lena Tabori
the mother

Looking Back

Making the decision to have
a child–it's momentous.
It is to decide forever to
have your heart go walking
around outside your body.
—*Elizabeth Stone*

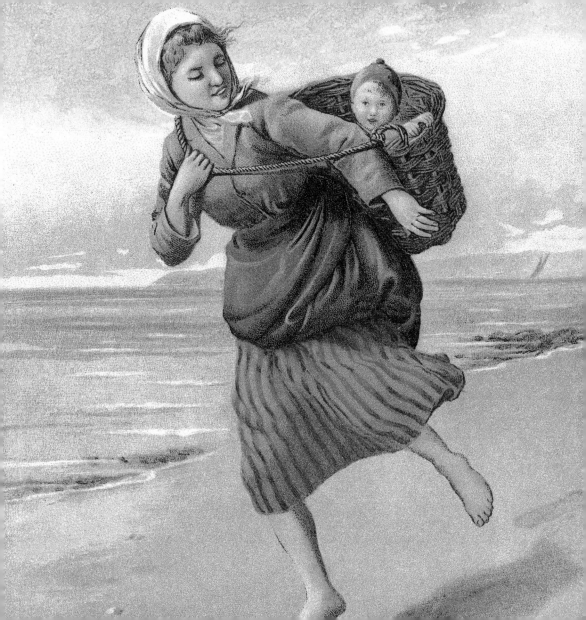

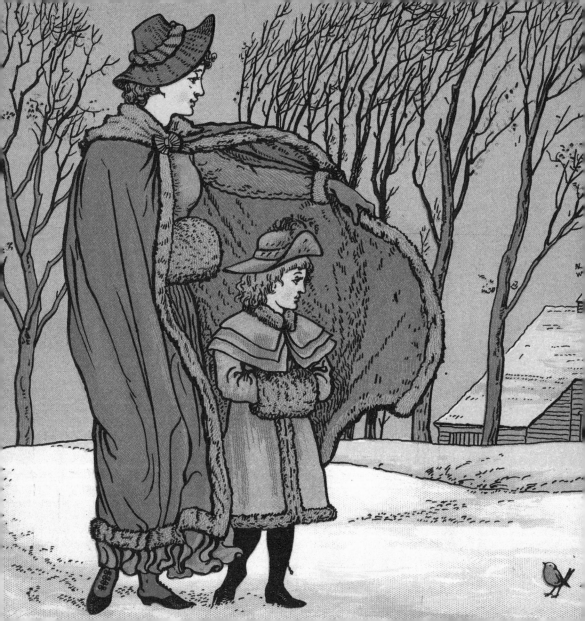

For Mothers and Future Mothers

Dale Hanson Bourke

WE ARE SITTING at lunch when my daughter casually mentions that she and her husband are thinking of "starting a family". "We're taking a survey," she says, half-joking. "Do you think I should have a baby?"

"It will change your life," I say, carefully keeping my tone neutral.

"I know," she says, "no more sleeping in on weekends, no more spontaneous vacations...."

But that is not what I meant at all. I look at my daughter, trying to decide what to tell her. I want her to know what she will never learn in childbirth classes. I want to tell her that the physical wounds of child bearing will heal, but that becoming a mother will leave her with an emotional wound so raw that she will forever be vulnerable. I consider warning her that she will never again read a newspaper without asking "What if that had been MY child?" That every plane crash, every house fire will haunt her. That when she sees pictures of starving children, she will wonder if anything could be worse than watching your child die.

I look at her carefully manicured nails and stylish suit and think that no matter how sophisticated she is, becoming a mother will reduce her to the primitive level of a bear protecting her cub. That an urgent call of "Mom!" will cause her to drop a souffle or her best crystal without a moment's hesitation.

I feel I should warn her that no matter how many years she has invested in her career, she will be professionally derailed by motherhood. She might arrange for childcare, but one day she will be going into an important business meeting and she will think of her baby's sweet smell. She will have to use every ounce of her discipline to keep from running home, just to make sure her baby is all right.

I want my daughter to know that everyday decisions will no longer be routine. That a five year old boy's desire to go to the men's room rather than the women's at McDonald's will become a major dilemma. That right there, in the midst of clattering trays and screaming children, issues of independence and gender identity will be weighed against the prospect that a child molester may be lurking in that restroom.

However decisive she may be at the office, she will second-guess herself constantly as a mother.

Looking at my attractive daughter, I want to assure her that eventually she will shed the pounds of pregnancy, but she will never feel the same about herself. That her life, now so important, will be of less value to her once she has a child. That she would give it up in a moment to save her offspring, but will also begin to hope for more years—not to accomplish her own dreams, but to watch her child accomplish theirs.

For Mothers and Future Mothers

I want her to know that a cesarean scar or shiny stretch marks will become badges of honor. My daughter's relationship with her husband will change, but not in the way she thinks. I wish she could understand how much more you can love a man who is careful to powder the baby or who never hesitates to play with his child. I think she should know that she will fall in love with him again for reasons she would now find very unromantic.

I wish my daughter could sense the bond she will feel with women throughout history who have tried to stop war, prejudice and drunk driving.

I hope she will understand why I can think rationally about most issues, but become temporarily insane when I discuss the threat of nuclear war to my children's future.

I want to describe to my daughter the exhilaration of seeing your child learn to ride a bike. I want to capture for her the belly laugh of a baby who is touching the soft fur of a dog or a cat for the first time. I want her to taste the joy that is so real, it actually hurts.

My daughter's quizzical look makes me realize that tears have formed in my eyes. "You'll never regret it," I finally say. Then I reach across the table, squeeze my daughter's hand and offer a silent prayer for her, and for me, and for all of the mere mortal women who stumble their way into this most wonderful of callings. This blessed gift from God...that of being a Mother.

Baby on the Way

Thinking back, what made you first think you were pregnant? Did you have trouble concentrating? Were you unusually tired? Emotional? Nauseated? "Late"? Before the days of fertility drugs and pregnancy tests, women had little more than their hopes and intuition to work with. Or did they? Throughout history, people have tried to encourage and predict conception. Read on and judge some of the more old-fashioned methods for yourself.

The Celtic Druids gathered acorns and carried pine cones to promote fertility. In some parts of ancient England, Germany, and Scandinavia where oak trees were said to be favored by the Norse god Thor, acorns also were considered to be totems of sexual power. The Romans and Greeks carried flowers and herbs to protect against illness and encourage fertility. Other traditional fertility talismans include horseshoes and the more well-known mistletoe.

Wedding ceremonies have long been rich with fertility rites. Wedding cakes supposedly began as the sweet cakes of Roman times which were

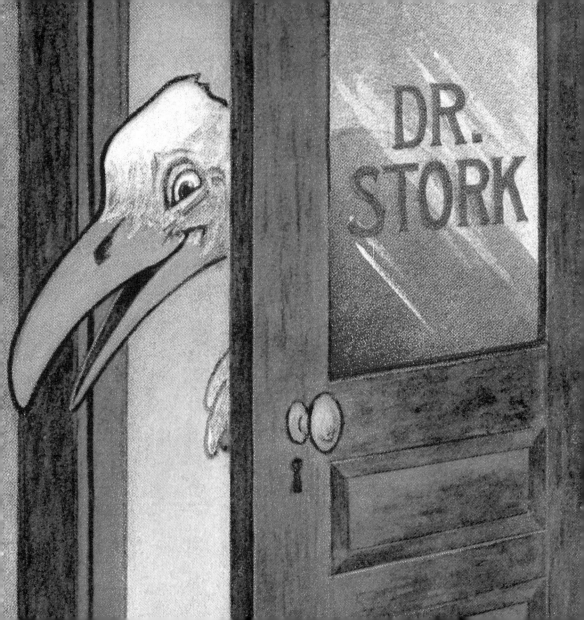

thought to bring fertility, happiness, and abundance. Ever wonder why you throw rice at a new bride and groom? Some say the tradition began as guests throwing bits of the wedding cake, or by crumbling bread over the couple's heads, or by showering the couple with wheat or corn. But whatever its origin, the throwing of grain—a symbol of bountiful harvests—is clearly meant to encourage fertility. Even sprays of baby's breath, now a common element of the bridal bouquet, began as fertility symbols.

Newlyweds have always been swamped with baby expectations. An American folktale says that stuffing garlic in the keyhole of your honeymoon-suite door ensures a quick pregnancy. Another eastern European fertility custom is said to be the origin of the "cat's cradle." Cats were often considered symbols of fertility, and after a wedding, a cat was put in a cradle and taken to the newlyweds' house. For a sure-fire, speedy conception, the cat was then rocked in the couple's presence.

Many traditions and superstitions surround the prediction of childbirth as well. Jewish scholars wrote that if a man dreamed of a vineyard, of sleeping under trees, or of carrying a bird in his bosom it foretold of future children. Others believe that baby dreams mean a child will be born into your family. Fish dreams suggest someone you know is pregnant.

If you have trouble sleeping, take a peek out your window. A bright star predicts that someone will soon give birth. If your right eye starts to twitch, that's the sign of an imminent birth in your family. In the morning, you might look for a rainbow. On the Orkney Islands (off Scotland), a bright rainbow preceded the birth of a boy. If you're distracted by a rabbit running across your yard, know that the bounding bunny means that this year will be a good time to have children. And if you're getting dressed and realize you've lost a pair of earrings, a Guatemalan folktale asserts you will surely become pregnant within six short months.

Of course, many beliefs center on babies themselves. If a married woman is the first to see a newborn, she will be the next to have a baby. A woman who holds an infant on her first visit to a new mother will soon be a mother too. Find a baby's pacifier and your family can expect a baby soon. And a wives' tale version of Murphy's Law warns that giving away outgrown baby clothes will mean you'll inevitably need them again soon.

Our last tale sounds like an assertion any astute, overprotective mother might rally behind. Rumor has it that a woman who lays her hat or coat on an unfamiliar bed will soon become pregnant. Hmmm…wonder where the Old Wives got that idea?

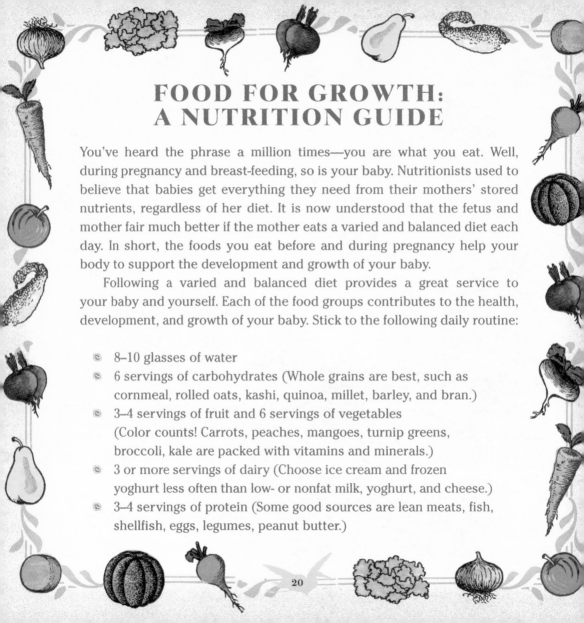

FOOD FOR GROWTH:
A NUTRITION GUIDE

You've heard the phrase a million times—you are what you eat. Well, during pregnancy and breast-feeding, so is your baby. Nutritionists used to believe that babies get everything they need from their mothers' stored nutrients, regardless of her diet. It is now understood that the fetus and mother fair much better if the mother eats a varied and balanced diet each day. In short, the foods you eat before and during pregnancy help your body to support the development and growth of your baby.

Following a varied and balanced diet provides a great service to your baby and yourself. Each of the food groups contributes to the health, development, and growth of your baby. Stick to the following daily routine:

- 8–10 glasses of water
- 6 servings of carbohydrates (Whole grains are best, such as cornmeal, rolled oats, kashi, quinoa, millet, barley, and bran.)
- 3–4 servings of fruit and 6 servings of vegetables (Color counts! Carrots, peaches, mangoes, turnip greens, broccoli, kale are packed with vitamins and minerals.)
- 3 or more servings of dairy (Choose ice cream and frozen yoghurt less often than low- or nonfat milk, yoghurt, and cheese.)
- 3–4 servings of protein (Some good sources are lean meats, fish, shellfish, eggs, legumes, peanut butter.)

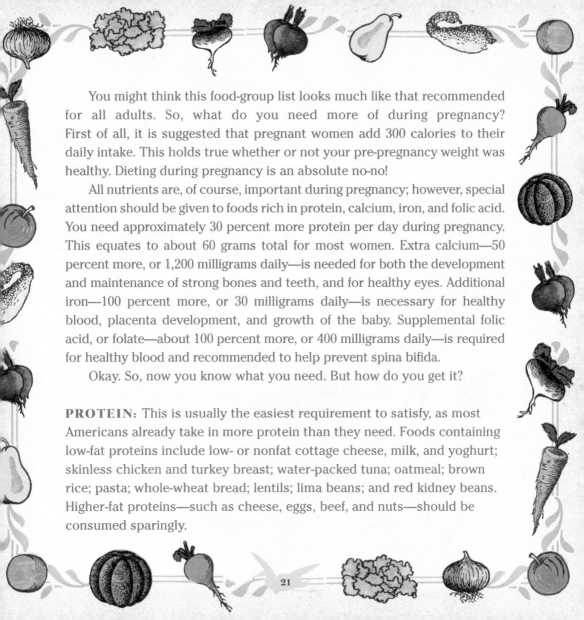

You might think this food-group list looks much like that recommended for all adults. So, what do you need more of during pregnancy? First of all, it is suggested that pregnant women add 300 calories to their daily intake. This holds true whether or not your pre-pregnancy weight was healthy. Dieting during pregnancy is an absolute no-no!

All nutrients are, of course, important during pregnancy; however, special attention should be given to foods rich in protein, calcium, iron, and folic acid. You need approximately 30 percent more protein per day during pregnancy. This equates to about 60 grams total for most women. Extra calcium—50 percent more, or 1,200 milligrams daily—is needed for both the development and maintenance of strong bones and teeth, and for healthy eyes. Additional iron—100 percent more, or 30 milligrams daily—is necessary for healthy blood, placenta development, and growth of the baby. Supplemental folic acid, or folate—about 100 percent more, or 400 milligrams daily—is required for healthy blood and recommended to help prevent spina bifida.

Okay. So, now you know what you need. But how do you get it?

PROTEIN: This is usually the easiest requirement to satisfy, as most Americans already take in more protein than they need. Foods containing low-fat proteins include low- or nonfat cottage cheese, milk, and yoghurt; skinless chicken and turkey breast; water-packed tuna; oatmeal; brown rice; pasta; whole-wheat bread; lentils; lima beans; and red kidney beans. Higher-fat proteins—such as cheese, eggs, beef, and nuts—should be consumed sparingly.

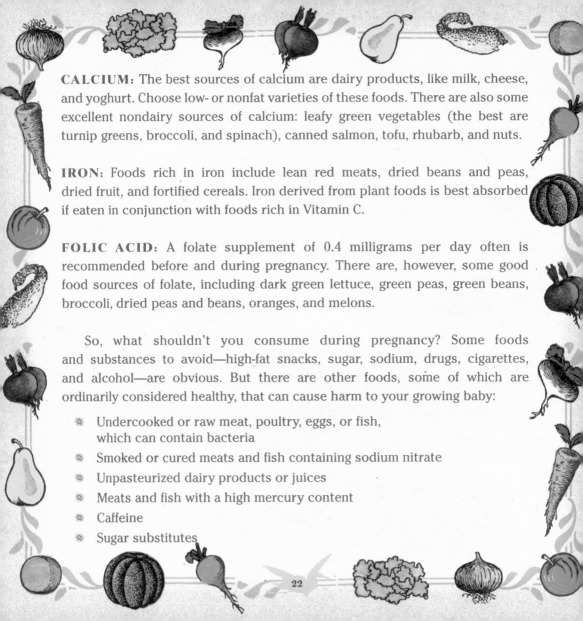

CALCIUM: The best sources of calcium are dairy products, like milk, cheese, and yoghurt. Choose low- or nonfat varieties of these foods. There are also some excellent nondairy sources of calcium: leafy green vegetables (the best are turnip greens, broccoli, and spinach), canned salmon, tofu, rhubarb, and nuts.

IRON: Foods rich in iron include lean red meats, dried beans and peas, dried fruit, and fortified cereals. Iron derived from plant foods is best absorbed if eaten in conjunction with foods rich in Vitamin C.

FOLIC ACID: A folate supplement of 0.4 milligrams per day often is recommended before and during pregnancy. There are, however, some good food sources of folate, including dark green lettuce, green peas, green beans, broccoli, dried peas and beans, oranges, and melons.

So, what shouldn't you consume during pregnancy? Some foods and substances to avoid—high-fat snacks, sugar, sodium, drugs, cigarettes, and alcohol—are obvious. But there are other foods, some of which are ordinarily considered healthy, that can cause harm to your growing baby:

- Undercooked or raw meat, poultry, eggs, or fish, which can contain bacteria
- Smoked or cured meats and fish containing sodium nitrate
- Unpasteurized dairy products or juices
- Meats and fish with a high mercury content
- Caffeine
- Sugar substitutes

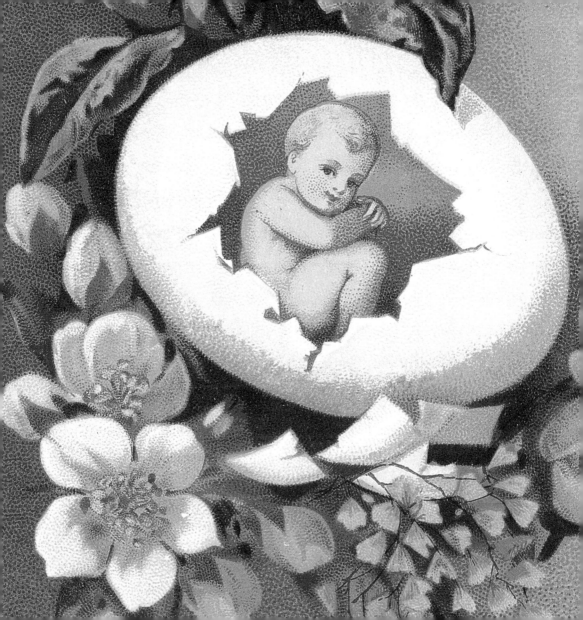

Why, when I was told the news,
I felt wings upon my shoes
And gallivanted down the street
Wanting to be indiscreet
And shout to all the world that
I
Was about to multiply.

–*Dorothy Keeley Aldis*

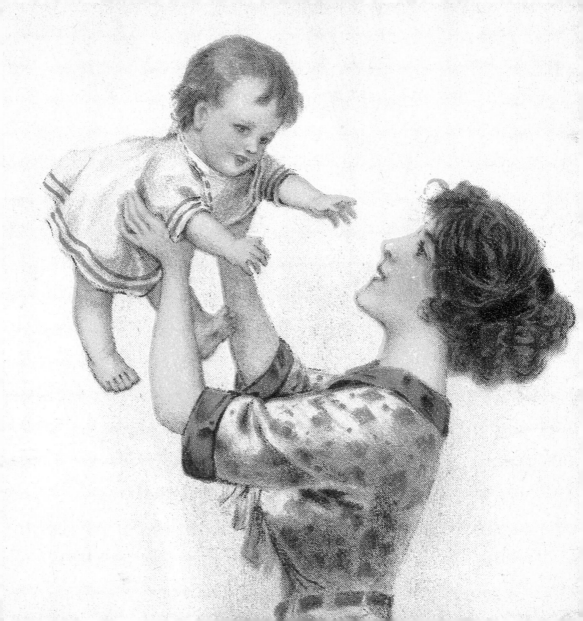

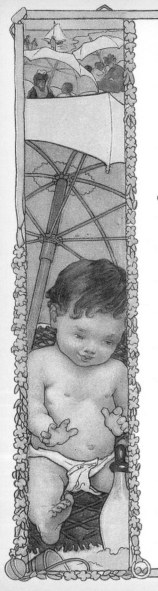

PREGNANCY FACTS

The salty fluid inside the amniotic sac protects the embryo not only from shocks, but from gravity as well. To see how this works, drop an egg still in the shell into a mayonnaise jar full of water, and shake it around.

On the 22nd day after conception the baby develops a heartbeat.

At the end of the first month of pregnancy, the baby is smaller than a grain of rice.

During pregnancy, a woman's blood volume increases nearly 50 percent.

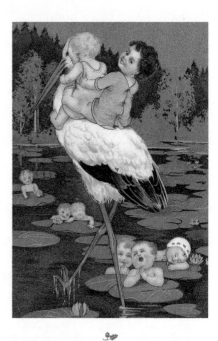

During the course of a typical pregnancy, a woman's uterus will expand up to 20 times its normal size.

In the womb, amniotic fluid is completely recirculated by the baby every three hours.

By the ninth week, the head comprises about half of the fetus, but its growth will now slow down compared to the rest of the body.

By the 18th week in utero, a female fetus has her own fully formed uterus.

At 36 weeks, the baby is storing fat—which keeps him or her at about 32°F above the mother's body temperature.

By seven months of age, a fetus can recognize his/her mother's voice.

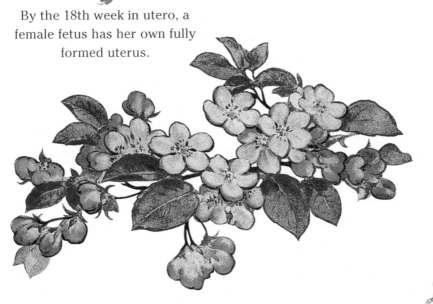

Prodigal Summer

Barbara Kingsolver

FOR THE REST OF HER OWN LIFE and maybe the next one after, Deanna would remember this day. A cool snap had put a sudden premonition of fall into the air, a crisp quality she could feel with her skin and all the rest of her newly heightened senses: she could smell and taste the change, even hear it. The birds had gone quiet, their noisy summer celebration hushed all at once by the power of a cold front and the urge rising up in their breasts to be still, gather in, wait for the time soon to come when they would turn in the darkness on a map made of stars and join the vast assembly of migration. Deanna clung to her perch on the rock, feeling the same stirring in her breast, a sense of finished business and a longing to fly. She had climbed up onto a lichen-crusted boulder fifty feet above the spot where the trail ended at the overlook. From here she could look down on everything, the valley of her childhood and the mountains beyond it. If she stood and spread her arms, it seemed possible she would sail out beyond everything she'd yet known, into new territory.

From the branches behind her she heard a sociable gathering of friends hailing each other with their winter call: chicka *dee-dee-dee!*

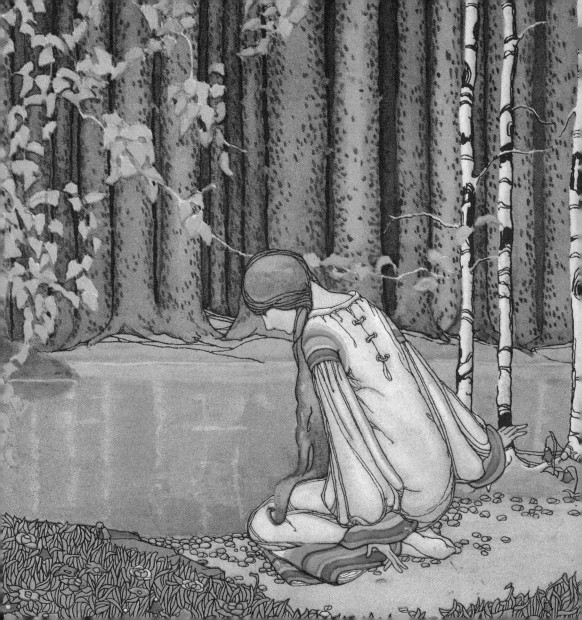

Prodigal Summer

The chickadees, her familiar anchors. Deanna would not fly away today; this thrill was only something left over from childhood, when a crisp turn in the weather meant apple time, time to hunt for paw-paws in Nannie's woodlot. At some point between yesterday and today the air had gone from soggy to brittle. The Virginia creeper on the cabin had begun to turn overnight; this morning she'd noticed a few bright-red leaves, just enough to make her pause and take note of history. This was the day, would always be the day, when she first knew. She would step somehow from the realm of ghosts that she'd inhabited all her life to commit herself irrevocably to the living. On the trail up to this overlook today she had paid little mind to the sadness of lost things moving through the leaves at the edges of her vision, the shadowy little wolves and the bright-winged parakeets hopping wistfully through untouched cockleburs. These dispossessed creatures were beside her and always would be, but just for today she noticed instead a single bright-red berry among all the clusters of green ones covering the spicebushes. This sign seemed meaningful and wondrous, standing as a divide between one epoch of her life and the next. If the summer had to end somewhere, why couldn't it be in that one red spicebush berry beside the path?

She slipped the small, borrowed mirror—his shaving mirror— from her back pocket and looked closely at her face. With the fingertips of her left hand she touched the slightly mottled, darker skin beneath her eyes. It was like a raccoon's mask, but subtler, spreading from the bridge of her nose out to her cheekbones. The rest of her face was the same as she remembered it, unmoved if not untouched. Her breasts were heavier; she could feel that change internally. She turned her face to the sun and slowly unbuttoned her shirt, placing his hands like ghost fingers where hers were now. His touch on her skin would be a mantle she could shed and put on again through the power of memory. Here on this rock in the sun she let him enter her like water: the memory of this morning, his eyes in hers, his movement like a tide pushing the sea against the sand of its only shore. Her body's joy was colored darker now from knowing that each conversation, every kiss, every comforting adventure of skin on skin might be the last one. Each image stood still beside its own shadow. Even the warmth of his body sleeping next to her afterward was a dark-brown heat she stroked with her fingers, memorizing it against the days when that space would be cold.

Fifty feet below her was the overlook where she'd nearly ended her life in a fall two years ago, and then, in May, where she'd fallen again. *Sweet*, he'd said. *Did you ever see a prettier sight than that right there?* And she'd replied, Never. She was looking at mountains and valleys, all keeping their animal secrets. He was looking at sheep farms.

Prodigal Summer

She touched her breast and took up the mirror again to look closely at the deep auburn color of her aureole. It seemed like a miracle that skin could change like this in color and texture in such a short time, like caterpillar skin taking on the color and texture of moth. Briefly, as if testing the temperature of water, she touched her abdomen just under her navel, where the top button of her jeans no longer conceded to meet its buttonhole. Deanna wondered briefly just how much of a fool she had been, for how long. Ten weeks at the most, probably less, but *still*. She'd known bodies, her own especially, and she hadn't known this. Was it something a girl learned from a mother, that secret church of female knowledge that had never let her in? All the things she'd heard women say did not seem right. She had not been sick, had not craved to eat anything strange. (Except for a turkey. Was that strange?) She'd only felt like a bomb had exploded in the part of her mind that kept her on an even keel. She'd mistaken that feeling for love or lust or peri-menopause or an acute invasion of privacy, and as it turned out it was all of those, and none. The explosion had frightened her for the way it loosened her grip on the person she'd always presumed herself to be. But maybe that was what this was going to be: a long, long process of coming undone from one's self.

Contrary to myth, no culture is immune to the "joys" of morning sickness. Papyrus texts show people understood unexpected nausea as far back as 2000 B.C. Women and caregivers, from the African !Kung San tribe to the Greek physician Hippocrates, have long recognized morning sickness as one of pregnancy's earliest signs.

While it often strikes at dawn, morning sickness is in no way confined to the morning. Most non-Westerners don't even use "morning" to describe the symptoms. Cantonese expectant mothers have a "pregnancy response." Russians display a "pregnancy indisposition." And in Korea, pregnant women simply enjoy "fake vomiting."

Whatever the name, 60–80 percent of all pregnant women experience strong food, drink, and smell aversions and/or vomiting, typically from week 4 through week 12. The cause is still unclear: Some believe the symptoms stem from an increase in pregnancy hormones, low blood sugar, or higher bile secretion. Others think the food and smell aversions actually serve a biological purpose, protecting the developing baby by discouraging the mom from ingesting harmful plants and toxins.

Home Remedies: *Morning Sickness*

But knowing the cause won't settle your stomach; so treat yourself to some of our soothing home remedies. Experiment. See what works for you. And remember, Old Wives' tales are told by women who survived pregnancy and lived to be chatty Old Wives!

(Note: If you vomit excessively, always call your caregiver. Dehydration can be dangerous to you *and* your baby!)

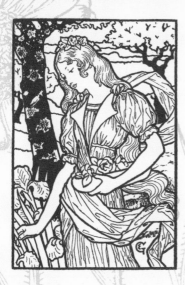

Rest & Exercise

- Try closing your eyes and lying completely still.
- Take naps, but not immediately after meals.
- Get out of bed slowly in the morning.
- Experiment with deep breathing and relaxation exercises.
- Sit and stand up straight.
- Take a walk at least once a day.
- Avoid making quick movements.

Meals & Snacks

- Eat small, frequent, high-protein, high-carbohydrate, low-fat meals. Fatty foods take longer to digest, promoting nausea.
- Eat crackers and breads made of whole grain.
- Try crunchy, salty foods.
- Avoid greasy, spicy, or smelly foods.
- If vomiting persists, try sticking with one food you know you can tolerate. Add another food each day, as your stomach allows.
- Eat whatever you can keep down whenever you want it. Better to eat less than ideally than not gain the needed weight.
- Keep a snack by your bed to eat before you get up.
- Always keep a little food in your stomach; nausea occurs more frequently on an empty stomach.
- Snack often on dry, high-carbohydrate foods (crackers, vanilla wafers, toast, cereals). They go down easily and stay down.
- Try frozen popsicles, fruit sorbets, ice cream, yoghurt, or milk shakes.

Drinks

- 🌱 Drink between, instead of with, meals.
- 🌱 Drink small amounts of fluids regularly to avoid dehydration—up to 12 glasses a day.
- 🌱 Drink non-caffeinated teas, like peppermint, ginger root, and chamomile.
- 🌱 Try room-temperature drinks or "flat" sodas.
- 🌱 Try sucking on ice chips.
- 🌱 Try milk sweetened with sugar or pasteurized honey.
- 🌱 Dissolve wheat germ in warm milk; try sipping a few teaspoons hourly.

Herbs/Supplements

(Always consult your caregiver before trying any of these!)

- 🌱 Suck on peppermint candies. Be sure candy is made with real peppermint oil and not artificial flavoring.
- 🌱 Try taking your prenatal vitamins later in the day (or talk to your caregiver about temporarily stopping your prenatals to see if nausea eases; you may still need to take folic acid.)
- 🌱 Talk to your caregiver about changing your iron supplement. Iron can be rough on your stomach..

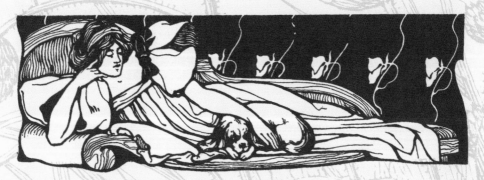

Aromatherapy

- Sniff a fresh lemon peel.

- Drip 3 drops lavender oil and 1 drop peppermint oil into a diffuser to freshen the air.

- Put a cool, lavender-scented cloth on your forehead and a warm lavender compress over your chest.

- Make sure you breathe as much fresh air as possible.

Triggers

(If reading this makes you sick, skip it!)

- Avoid strong odors, like coffee, fish, onions, garlic, garbage, vitamins, perfume, cigarette smoke, dirty diapers, gas fumes, room fresheners, and cleaning products.

- If you can't escape a noxious smell, breathe through a tissue pre-dipped in a non-nauseating essential oil such as lemon, grapefruit, ginger, or spearmint.

- Turn on fans and open windows when you cook.

- Cook with a microwave to minimize smells.

- Avoid cooking by eating prepackaged meals.

- Try eating more cold foods; they often have less nauseating odors.

- Tank up at full-service gas stations.

Some Other Good Ideas

- Don't brush your teeth right after a meal.

- Wear motion sickness wristbands to stimulate acupressure points.

- Try meditation and yoga to relax your mind and body.

- Try chewing gum.

- Stay away from warm places; higher temperatures can increase nausea.

Foetal Song

Joyce Carol Oates

The vehicle gives a lurch but seems
to know its destination.
In here, antique darkness. I guess at things.
Tremors of muscles communicate
secrets to me. I am nourished.
A surge of blood pounding sweet
blossoms my gentle head.
I am perfumed wax melted of holy candles
I am ready to be fingered and shaped.
This cave unfolds to my nudge, which
seems gentle but is hard as steel.
Coils of infinite steel are my secret.
Within this shadowless cave I am not confused
I think I am a fish, or a small seal.
I have an impulse to swim, but without
moving; *she* moves and I drift after . . .
I am a trout silent and gilled, a tiny seal
a slippery monster knowing all secrets.
Where is she off to now?–in high heels.
I don't like the jiggle of high heels.

On the street we hear horns, drills, feel sleeves,
feel rushes of language moving by
and every stranger has possibly
my father's face.

Now we are in bed.
Her heart breathes quiet and I drink blood.
I am juicy and sweet and coiled.
Her dreams creep upon me through nightmare
    slots of windows
I cringe from them, unready.
I don't like such pictures.
Morning...and the safety of the day brings us
bedroom slippers, good.
Day at home, comfort in this sac,
three months from my birthday I dream
upon songs and eerie music, angels' flutes
that tear so stern upon earthly anger
(now they are arguing again).
Jokes and unjokes, married couple,

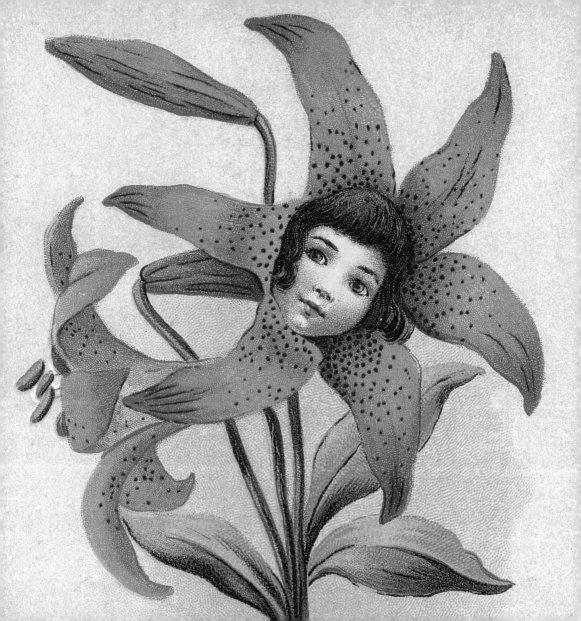

they clutch at each other in water
I feel him nudge me but it is by accident.
The darkness of their sacs must be slimy with dead tides
and hide what they knew of ponds and knotty ropes of lilies.
It forsakes them now, cast into the same bed.
The tide throws them relentlessly into the same bed.
While he speaks to her I suck marrow from her bones.
It has a grainy white taste, a little salty.
Oxygen from her tremendous lungs taste white too
but airy bubbles, it makes me dizzy...!

She speaks to him and her words do not matter.
Marrow and oxygen matter eternally. They are mine.
Sometimes she walks on concrete, my vehicle,
sometimes on gravel, on grass, on the
blank worn tides of our floors at home.
She and he, months ago, decided not to kill me.
I rise and fall now like seaweed fleshed to fish, a surprise.
I am grateful.
I am waiting for my turn.

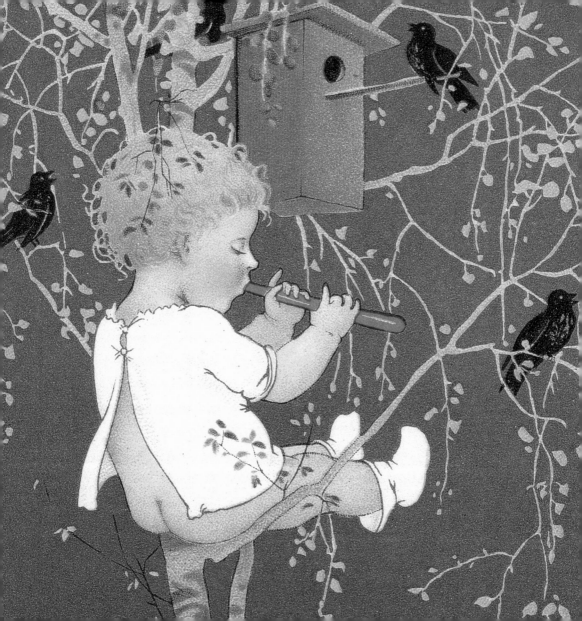

TRADITIONS: *Music & Lullabies*

Music has forever been a part of our joyous occasions and celebrations. In many cultures, it plays a pivotal role in pregnancy, birth, and child rearing. Western authorities on the subject often recommend playing classical melodies to stimulate your unborn baby and shorten labor.

In India during a Parsi ritual called *Agharni*, which takes place after the seventh month of pregnancy, relatives gather to worship, present gifts, and sing to the mother-to-be. Navaho medicine people traditionally chant and, when necessary, sing "unraveling" songs to help with labor and coax the baby out. A long-held belief by Englanders purports that the ringing of church bells helps to ease a baby's birth. A call-and-response song used in the Central African Republic during delivery goes, *Ei-oh mother of mine, my belly hurts me.* The response is *Tie up your heart*, which means "Tough it out." After a baby is born in Morocco, women and children "sing the news," proclaiming to all the new birth. And in Latvia, after the baby's naming ceremony, guests and godparents attend a feast, dancing with the baby and singing songs of good wishes.

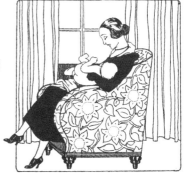

A favorite form of music the world over is the lullaby; a simple, gentle, often repetitive song that parents croon while rocking their little ones to sleep. Lullabies reassure children that everything is all right, that they are loved and cared for, and that their parents are close at hand. Some lullabies express parents' hopes and worries. Others tell stories and teach lessons. Hushed lullabies sung by the Mossi of Burkina Faso tell the baby of his or her family history, musically passing along the entire family tree.

We've gathered together some much beloved lullabies from around the world. Read through them, if only to remember the words of a favorite from childhood. Many mothers enjoy singing to their little one in the womb. And later, if you can't remember every verse, don't stop singing. Rock your baby and hum. Your loving, soothing voice is often comfort enough.

CAROLINE ISLANDS, ULITHI ATOLL
Float on the water,
In my arms, my arms,
On the little sea,
On the big sea,
The channel sea,
The rough sea,
The calm sea,
On this sea.

FRANCE
Are you sleeping, are you sleeping?
Brother John, Brother John?
Morning bells are ringing, morning bells
    are ringing
Ding ding dong, ding ding dong.

GERMANY
(JOHANNES BRAHMS)

Lullaby and good night,
  with roses bedight
With lilies o'er spread
  is baby's wee bed
Lay thee down now and rest,
  may thy slumber be blessed
Lay thee down now and rest,
  may thy slumber be blessed.

Lullaby and good night,
  thy mother's delight
Bright angels beside
  my darling abide
They will guard thee at rest, thou
  shalt wake on my breast
They will guard thee at rest, thou
  shalt wake on my breast

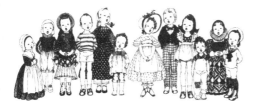

GREECE

Now then sleep, sleep my child.
Sleep and dream my lovely child.
I'll give you the city of
Alexandria in sugar;
All of Cairo in rice.
And rich Constantinople.
And there you shall reign for
three years.

HAITI

Sleep mosquitoes sleep,
Sleep mosquitoes sleep.
Three hours before dawn
Mosquitoes begin to sting
I know not which position
To shift to!
Sleep mosquitoes sleep.

HOPI

Pu'va, pu'va, pu'va.
On the trail the beetles
On each others' backs are sleeping.

So on mine my baby, thou.
Pu'va, pu'va, pu'va.
Pu'va, pu'va, pu'va.

IRELAND

Over in Killarney
Many years ago
Me mother sang a song to me
In tones so sweet and low.
Just a simple little ditty,
In her good old Irish way,
And I'd give the world
If she could sing
That song to me this day.

Too-ra-loo-ra-loo-ra
Too-ra-loo-ra-li
Too-rà-loo-ra-loo-ra
Hush now don't you cry
Too-ra-loo-ra-loo-ra
Too-ra-loo-ra-li
Too-ra-loo-ra-loo-ra
That's an Irish lullaby.

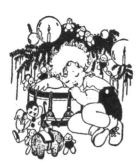

RUSSIA

Sleep, ah sleep, my darling baby,
Su, su, lullaby.
See the moon is watching o'er thee,
Peacefully on high.
Thou shalt hear a wondrous story,
Close each wakeful eye,
And a song as well I'll sing thee,
Su, su, lullaby.

USA

Hush little baby, don't say a word.
Papa's gonna buy you a mockingbird.
And if that mockingbird won't sing,
Papa's gonna buy you a diamond
    ring.
And if that diamond ring turns brass,
Papa's gonna buy you a looking
    glass.
And if that looking glass gets broke,
Papa's gonna buy you a billy goat.
And if that billy goat won't pull,
Papa's gonna buy you a cart and bull.
And if that cart and bull fall down,
You'll still be the sweetest little baby
    in town.

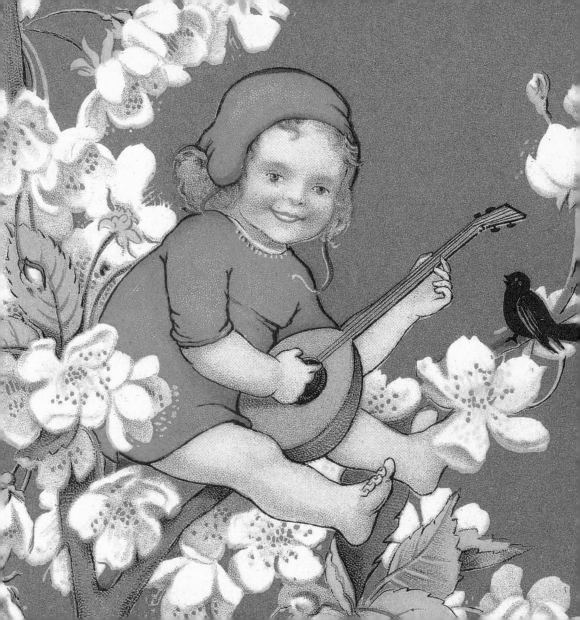

BABY HOROSCOPES

O
ne of the best parts of being pregnant is imagining who that little life inside you will turn out to be. Will she be a dancer, a doctor, a musician, a teacher? Will he be witty, wild, sensitive, or serious? How about ambitious or introspective? Well, we can't give you all the answers, but we did consult the stars, and here is what they have to say....

CAPRICORN

Your child is blessed with innate wisdom beyond experience, a love of competition, and a self-deprecating sense of humor. Your bundle of joy can excel in business and politics, and develops high personal standards. Lavish this baby with lots of love and praise to help balance self-effacing tendencies. Activity that evokes laughter helps lighten that serious nature.

AQUARIUS

Your life won't be dull, since the Aquarius child is full of surprises, and has been given the courage to be an individual in a world full of conformity. Aquarians are born to overthrow the past and invent the future, so this little one loves experimenting and testing limits. Nurture that innate curiosity and the rewards will be great for both parents and child.

PISCES

Tenderhearted, intuitive, creative, with boundless imagination and the soul of a poet, your Pisces child excels in work and play activities that utilize these wonderful gifts. Water and music soothes the spirit and nurtures talent too. Trying to shield this intuitive child from unpleasant emotions or experiences is impossible, so deliver the truth, tailored to suit his age.

ARIES

Get ready for the ride of your life—this little soul is a powerhouse of energy and talents. *Active* is the keyword, and *fearless* too, so remove tall objects once climbing is mastered or attach a bungee cord for safety's sake. Innate confidence and natural leadership abilities can lead to success in a myriad of fields. Discipline is needed, but not so firm that it breaks her spirit.

TAURUS

Your little Taurus is creative, naturally easygoing, and has great common sense. She loves soft fabrics and the touch of your hand. A baby massage soothes and satisfies a little Taurus's need for physical sensation; regular routines provide security; and a love of food and drink gives him a healthy appetite. Endurance and patience are assets that can turn to stubbornness in a test of wills.

GEMINI

Curiosity personified is your precious Gemini, along with a quick wit, imagination, and intellect. A fun-loving nature makes settling down to do one thing impossible, but her ability to juggle several activities at once is innate, so handling a variety of tasks later on will be second nature. *Changeable*, *adaptable*, and *versatile* are keywords to your child's talents and happiness.

CANCER

Cancer is *the* zodiac sign for childhood, family, and home, so feelings and nurturing instincts are strong here. You can never love a Cancer child too much or too often: Like a flower, he blooms or wilts, stands tall, or clings to the vine, depending on the love he receives. Mom and Dad are everything to this little soul, and the language of the heart is the one that Cancer knows best.

LEO

Mom and Dad have every right to be proud of their little Leo, who is blessed with a sunny disposition, loving heart, abundant creativity, and instinctual leadership abilities. A natural flair for drama is an asset that can serve her well in both business and the arts— perhaps even on stage or screen. Pride is strong too, along with Leo's innate dignity, so discipline in private and praise in public.

VIRGO

Keep your running shoes handy, because this child will be in constant motion, both physically *and* mentally. An active, curious mind coupled with unlimited nervous energy keeps parents on their toes. High personal standards, including a love of order and perfection, makes Virgo a little shy or self-deprecating, so your role is to reassure him with lots of love.

LIBRA

Born with natural grace and charm, this child has a winning way *and* appearance, being usually well proportioned and attractive, with an innate sense of style that can translate to success in the arts, especially fashion, design, and architecture. On the other hand, your peace-loving and fair-minded Libra could excel in law or public relations. Encourage decisiveness early and consistently.

SCORPIO

The intense little Scorpio will do nothing halfway. Intuitive and loyal, your child will bond deeply with loved ones, and can be possessive of people and property. Sharing is hard to learn but necessary and easier if a couple of toys are set aside solely for her use. Rejection is Scorpio's greatest fear, and love is the only antidote.

SAGITTARIUS

Optimistic, idealistic, and independent, your child is always looking for the next

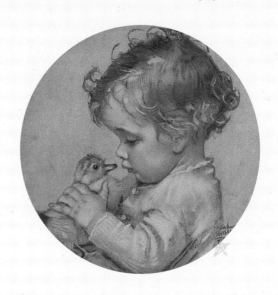

great adventure. Fun-loving and naturally athletic, he finds more activities and interests than there is time to do them. With age you'll see an above-average intellect and a dislike of routine or discipline. The Sagittarian child is blessed with a happy-go-lucky nature that will attract good will throughout her life.

Delusions of Grandma

Carrie Fisher

Dear Esme,

A LOT OF WHAT I DREADED about pregnancy are the things that actually occur. People squeal over you with delight. Strangers feel free to reach out and run their hands over the curve of your abdomen. It's as though because you have, in effect, lost control of your body, you have also lost control of your mind, causing people to emit loud noises when apprised of your maternal state. As though because you have been trespassed upon within, those without can feel free to rub you like some recently well worn rabbit's foot. I have taken a liking to the term *hysterical pregnancy*, though in my case the term's redundant. (Get it? Term/s redundant.)

I haven't had too many strange cravings, though. I think middle-of-the-night hankerings for pickles and ice cream was a notion popularized by James Garner films in the very early seventies. The only thing I've yearned for in the middle of the night is less indigestion and more sleep. I have, however, developed a real passion for cottage cheese, yogurt, milk, string cheese, and other high-cholesterol snack items. And, let's face it, I have a carnivorous inclination that is satisfied by drive-through—the only way I can

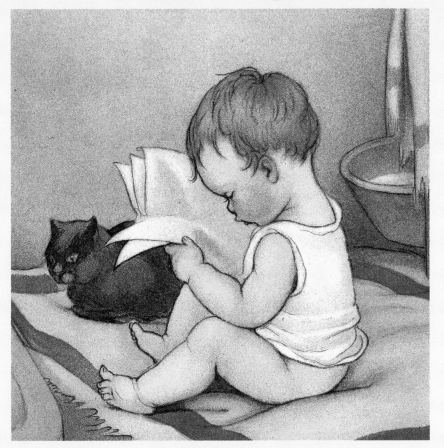
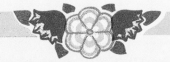

obtain food without waddling conspicuously through folks far less weight-ridden than myself.

I am doing a lot of driving and swimming—the only activities, as far as I can make out, that make me feel virtually weightless. The great thing about driving is that, in addition to feeling weightless as I skim over the asphalt, I feel powerful and defiant. I make my way through traffic, shrieking obscenities and giving the finger to male drivers (preferably in dangerous large trucks). So if one day you go into some sort of hypnosis and find yourself feeling whipped into a frenzy and ready for a brawl, it's not a past-life regression—it's simply you exercising your in-vitro invective on an assortment of men whom I blame for the more unpleasant aspects of my current state. In a fully estrogenized experience, it's nice to have the occasional testosterized triumph. I also plan for the birthing process to bring along a VCR and an assortment of Vietnam war documentaries, my reasoning being that childbirth is a female ritual in extremis, and war is a male ritual in extremis, and I am forever attempting to achieve a kind of balance where I can. Besides, I think it's important for you to have a taste of authentic androgen before it comes for a taste of you.

Being pregnant feels to me like a whale sounds, all mournful and down below. Flesh has collected on me like dust, like something left too long in a sealed room. Did you know that women have extra fat cells, to protect their unborn children? That is why men get craggy good looks that give them character as they get older, while we get the bleary, melted, overage-broad option. So enjoy your youth—or get a sex change (although I hear the technology is far from perfected).

In the meantime, everything grows rounder and wider and weirder, and I sit in the middle of it all and wonder who in the world you will turn out to be. I phoned an astrologer with your approximate date of arrival, and she said that if you were born on the tenth you would have dimples—on the twelfth, you wouldn't. She said that you would be very civic-minded and a good dresser, someone committed to saving endangered creatures and a talker to boot. I do not believe in astrology anyway. I was just checking.

Your motel,
Mom

Pregnancy Keepsake Diary

Create a record of these precious days and the events—big and small—that mark the progress of your pregnancy.

What To Do

◆ Buy a blank journal at the stationery or office supply store and assign each day of your pregnancy its own page.

◆ Write something down *every* day, even if it's just a single word that captures your mood, like GIDDY, FRUSTRATED, EXCITED, TIRED, HYPER, SEXY. Some days you'll have more to say, some days less. Or fill a page with a drawing or doodle—it's up to you.

◆ This diary should be *for your eyes only*, allowing you the freedom to write down your most intimate feelings. Record your dreams about the baby and being pregnant; vent about your aches, cravings, mood swings, and ballooning figure; revel in your fantasies about motherhood and the future of that little life inside you.

◆ Paste in small remembrances, such as your sonograms, your doctor's business card, photos of you and your partner during the pregnancy, scraps of gift paper from your shower, a chip of the paint you chose for the nursery, and anything else that has special meaning for you.

- On the practical side, your diary can also serve as an account of doctor visits, prenatal classes, the first time you feel the baby move, discovering the baby's sex, your baby shower, gifts you've received, belly measurements, favorite recipes, and name ideas.

- Consider sharing a passage every now and then with your partner, as long as you feel comfortable doing so. You may find it helps bring you closer together in the journey toward parenthood.

- Keep the diary somewhere safe and private. Visit it often in the years to come. You'll never tire of rereading its worn pages and reliving these precious days.

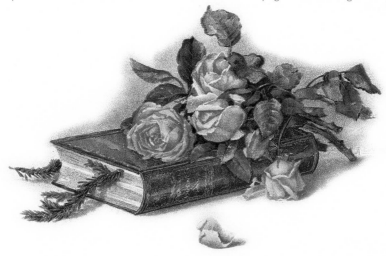

Letters to Your Unborn Child

Writing to your unborn child throughout your pregnancy is a wonderful way to nurture the developing bond between you and your baby. The experience of pregnancy brings with it a whole new set of emotions and perspectives that are unique to those very special nine months. Set aside a few hours each month to write a letter to the delicate life growing inside you. What to write is up to you. Imagine your son or daughter reading these letters decades from now and imagine what you'd like them know about this amazing period in your life together. Share your most memorable moments (what it felt like the first time you felt the baby kick), your hopes for the future (what you wish for your child's happiness), your fears (what scares you most about parenthood), your wisdom and advice (what you feel are life's most important lessons), or anything else that comes to mind. Write from your heart and give your child a gift that they will treasure for a lifetime.

What To Do

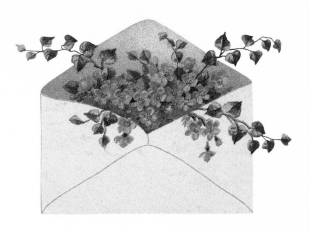

- Select a beautiful set of stationery.

- Set aside ten envelopes and label nine of them "Month 1" through "Month 9." Label the tenth envelope "Your Birth."

- Encourage your partner to include a letter each month as well. While they may not be experiencing the physical aspects of pregnancy, they too are preparing to become a parent.

- Once you have finished each letter, date it and seal it in the corresponding envelope. After your baby is born, write a final letter and include the birth story. Seal it in the last envelope, labeled "Your Birth."

- Place the envelopes in a plastic bag and store them in a sealed acid-free box. Address the box to your child and label it "Your First Nine Months."

- Store the box in a safe and dry place until the time arrives to give this special keepsake to your son or daughter. The occasion could be a momentous birthday, like sixteen or twenty-one, or a quiet, unplanned moment that simply presents itself. Regardless of the chosen time, it will certainly be received with surprise, gratitude, joy, and love.

Some Thoughts on Being Pregnant

Anne Lamott

THE SEVENTH AND EIGHTH GRADES were for me, and for every single good and interesting person I've ever known, what the writers of the Bible meant when they used the words *hell* and *the pit*. Seventh and eighth grades were a place into which one descended. One descended from the relative safety and wildness and bigness one felt in sixth grade, eleven years old. Then the worm turned, and it was all over for any small feeling that one was essentially all right. One wasn't. One was no longer just some kid. One was suddenly a Diane Arbus character. It was springtime, for Hitler, and Germany.

I experienced it as being a two-year game of "The farmer in the Dell." I hung out with the popular crowd, as jester, but boy, when those parties and dances rolled round, this cheese stood alone, watching my friends go steady and kiss, and then, like all you other cheeses, I went home and cried. There we were, all of us cheeses alone, emotionally broken by unrequited love and at the same time amped out of our minds on hormones and shame.

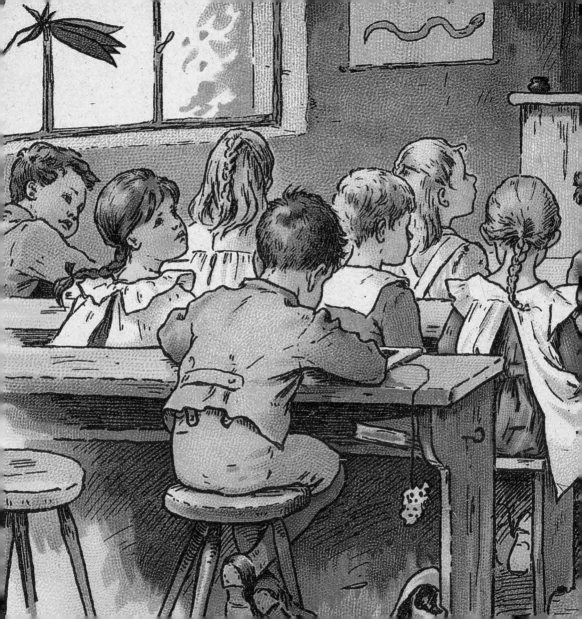

Some Thoughts on Being Pregnant

Seventh and eighth grades were about waiting to get picked for teams, waiting to get asked to dance, waiting to grow taller, waiting to grow breasts. They were about praying for God to grow dark hairs on my legs so I could shave them. They were about having pipe-cleaner legs. They were about violence, meanness, chaos. They were about *The Lord of the Flies*. They were about feeling completely other. But more than anything else, they were about hurt and aloneness. There is a beautiful poem by a man named Roy Fuller, which ends, "Hurt beyond hurting, never to forget," and whenever I remember those lines, which is often, I think of my father's death ten years ago this month, and I think about seventh and eighth grades.

So how on earth can I bring a child into the world, knowing that such sorrow lies ahead, that it is such a large part of what it means to be human?

I'm not sure. That's my answer: I'm not sure. One thing I do know is that I've recently been through it again, the total aloneness in the presence of almost extraterrestrially high levels of hormones. I have been thinking a lot lately of Phil Spector and his Wall of Sound, because to be pregnant is to be backed by a wall of hormones, just like during puberty, and the sense of aloneness that goes along with that is something I have been

Some Thoughts on Being Pregnant

dancing as fast as I could to avoid ever having to feel again. For the last twenty-some years, I have tried everything in sometimes suicidally vast quantities—alcohol, drugs, work, food, excitement, good deeds, popularity, men, exercise, and just rampant compulsion and obsession—to avoid having to be in the same room with that sense of total aloneness. And I did pretty well, although I nearly died. But then recently that aloneness walked right into my house without knocking, sat down, and stayed a couple of weeks.

In those two weeks, tremendous amounts of support poured in, as did baby clothes and furniture. My living room started to look like a refugee relocation center, but the aloneness was here, too, and it seemed to want to be felt. I was reminded once again that the people closest to me, including my therapist, function as my pit crew, helping me to fix blown-out tires and swabbing me off between laps, and the consensus, among those individuals who make up my pit crew, was that I was probably just going to have to go ahead and feel the aloneness for a while. So I did, and I'll tell you it didn't feel very good. But somehow I was finally able to stand in that huge open wound and feel it and acknowledge it because it was real, and the fear of the pain of this wound turned out to be worse than the actual pain.

Some Thoughts on Being Pregnant

As I said, though, it didn't feel very good, and it brought me up against that horrible, hateful truth—that there wasn't anything outside myself that could heal or fill me and that everything I had been running from and searching for all my life was within. So I sat with those things for a while, and the wounds began to heal.

This all took place a few months ago, at age thirty-five. I mean, I'm old and tough and I can take it. But Sam is just a baby. Sam, in fact, hasn't even come out of the chute yet. I guess when he does, there will be all these people to help him along on his journey; he will have his pit crews, too, but at some point he will also have to start seventh grade. Maybe he will be one of those kids who get off easy, but probably not. I don't know many who did. So he will find himself at some point, maybe many times, in what feels like a crawl space, scared of unseen spiders, pulling himself along on his elbows, the skin rubbed raw, not knowing for sure whether he will ever arrive at a place where he can stand up again in the daylight. This is what it feels like to grieve a loss that is just too big, the loss of a loved one, or of one's childhood, or whatever. (And it is sometimes what it feels like to be in the middle of writing a book; and also what it feels like sometimes when you've lost your hormonal equilibrium.)

Yet we almost always come out on the other side, maybe not with all our *f-a-c-u-l-t-i-e-s* intact, as Esmé put it, but in good enough shape. I was more or less okay by ninth grade. I am more or less okay now. I really love my pit crew, and I sometimes love my work. Sometimes it feels like God has reached down and touched me, blessed me a thousand times over, and sometimes it all feels like a mean joke, like God's advisers are Muammar Qaddafi and Phyllis Schlafly.

So I am often awake these days in the hours before the dawn, full of joy, full of fear. The first birds begin to sing at quarter after five, and when Sam moves around in my stomach, kicking, it feels like there are trout inside me, leaping, and I go in and out of the aloneness, in and out of that sacred place.

Often I am filled with hope; sometimes I am consumed with dread. Often I feel blessed; sometimes I feel resentful. Sometimes I am downright giddy. Sometimes I am so sentimental an AT&T commercial sends me over the edge. Sometimes I feel gorgeous, earthy, and powerful. Sometimes I feel like a helium balloon with gravity shoes...
A delusion, you say? Certainly not. Look, I'm not crazy—I'm pregnant.

—*Arlene Modica Matthews*

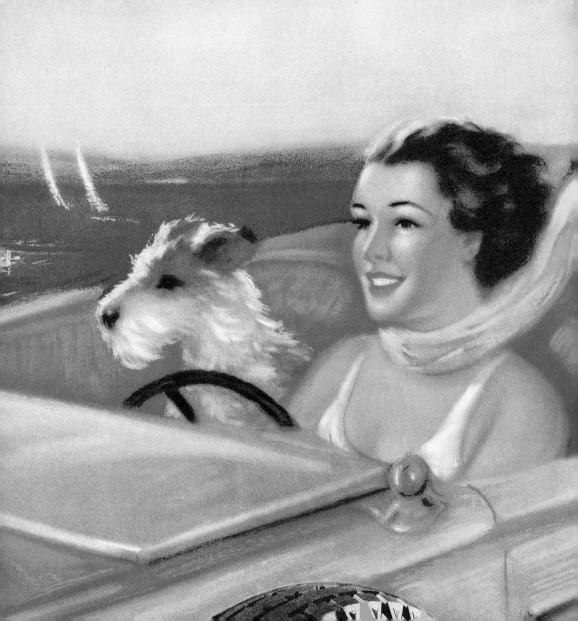

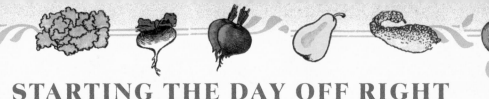

STARTING THE DAY OFF RIGHT

Some of us are seasoned breakfast skippers. But with a baby on the way, you just can't go without. Even morning sickness or a busy schedule is no excuse for missing your first meal of the day. So treat yourself and your baby to foods that are both scrumptious and healthy—you deserve it. Our friend Sara is due to have her baby any second, and she swears by the following breakfast treats.

ASPARAGUS FRITTATA

(Benefits: Served with fruit and whole-grain toast, this meal covers all the nutritional bases while giving you and your baby the extra protein and calcium you require. Be creative and use vegetables you have on hand to alter the recipe.)

Ingredients

1 ½ cups chopped asparagus
1 cup sliced mushrooms
1 scallion, chopped
1 garlic clove, minced
³/₄ teaspoon lemon juice
1 teaspoon chopped fresh thyme
4 eggs (substitute 1 egg and 5 egg whites to reduce cholesterol while retaining protein)
½ teaspoon kosher salt
½ cup water
½ cup low-fat milk
¼ cup Parmesan cheese, freshly grated

1. Preheat broiler.

2. Cook asparagus, mushrooms, scallion, and garlic in the lemon juice over medium heat until dry. Add thyme.

3. Whisk the eggs, salt, water, and milk together.

4. Remove the vegetable mixture from the heat and stir in the cheese.

5. Spray a large ovenproof skillet with light oil and heat on medium. Add the egg and vegetable mixtures to the skillet and cook until the eggs are set.

6. Place the skillet under the broiler; remove when top is lightly browned.

7. Divide between two warmed plates, and serve.

Serves 2.

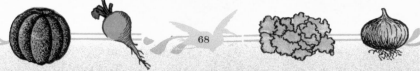

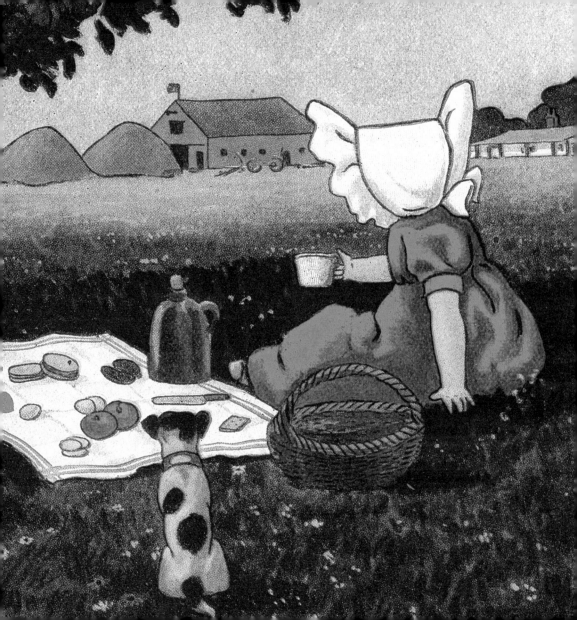

BLUEBERRY-BANANA OATMEAL MUFFINS

(Benefits: This low-fat, high-fiber muffin is a great alternative to its fatty counterparts. The banana and yoghurt make it moist and satisfying.)

Ingredients

1 cup rolled oats
1 cup whole-wheat flour
$^{1}/_{4}$ cup packed brown sugar
1 teaspoon baking powder
$^{1}/_{2}$ teaspoon baking soda
$^{1}/_{2}$ teaspoon ground cinnamon
$^{1}/_{4}$ teaspoon ground or freshly grated nutmeg
2 eggs
2 tablespoons vegetable oil
2 ripe bananas, mashed
1 cup plain nonfat yogurt
1 cup fresh or frozen blueberries

1. Preheat oven to 400 degrees.

2. Prepare muffin tins using paper liners or by greasing them with light oil or butter.

3. Grind the oats in an electric coffee grinder or crush them in a plastic bag with a rolling pin.

4. Sift all remaining dry ingredients into a large mixing bowl.

5. In another bowl, mix together all the wet ingredients and fruit.

6. Fold the wet mixture into the dry until lightly combined.

7. Spoon the batter into the muffin tins and bake for 20–25 minutes.

Makes 12 muffins.

LEMONY GINGERBREAD PANCAKES

(Benefits: The low sugar content of these yummy
pancakes spells good news for you and your baby!)

Ingredients

3 eggs

¹/₂ cup nonfat or low-fat milk

1 cup whole-wheat flour

¹/₄ cup sugar

2 teaspoons baking powder

¹/₂ teaspoon each ground ginger,
ground cinnamon,
and ground cloves

¹/₄ teaspoon ground or freshly
grated nutmeg

¹/₄ teaspoon kosher salt

1 tablespoon lemon zest

1. Whisk eggs and milk together in a
   small mixing bowl.

2. Sift dry ingredients together into a
   medium mixing bowl.

3. Fold wet mixture into dry until smooth.
   If the batter is too thick, add water
   as needed.

4. Heat griddle or large skillet over medium-
   high heat. Coat cooking area with cooking
   spray or margarine. Spoon ¹/₄ cup of
   batter at a time onto the heated surface
   and cook until bubbles form and remain
   open. Flip pancakes and brown the
   other side.

5. Place two pancakes each on warmed
   serving plates with applesauce or syrup.

Serves 4.

The Birth of the Water Baby

Erica Jong

Little egg,
little nub,
full complement of
fingers, toes,
little rose blooming
in a red universe,
which once wanted you less
than emptiness,
but now holds you
fast,
containing your rapid heart
beat under its
slower one
as the earth
contains the sea...

Oh avocado pit
almost ready to sprout,
tiny fruit tree
within sight
of the sea,

little swimming fish,
little land lover,
hold on!
hold on!

Here, under my heart
you'll keep
till it's time
for us to meet,
& we come apart
that we may come
together,
& you are born
remembering
the wavesound
of my blood,
the thunder of my heart,
& like your mother
always dreaming
of the sea.

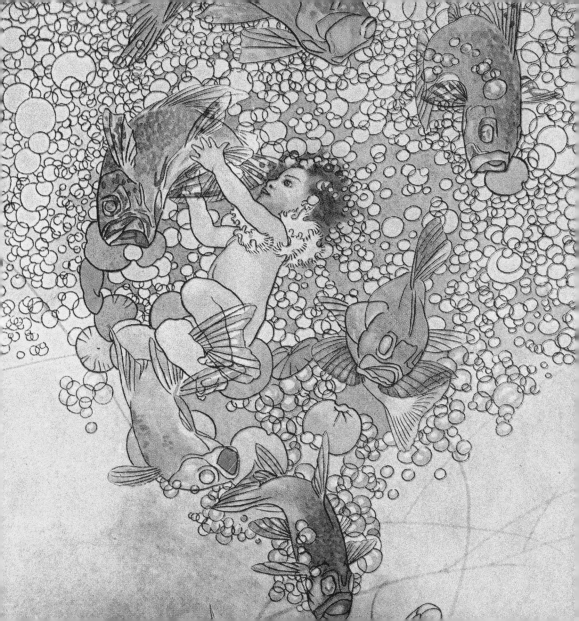

Midwives

Chris Bohjalian

BIRTH IS A BIG MIRACLE foreshadowed by lots of little ones. Conception. Little limbs. Lanugo. A fingerprint, hard bones. The quickening. The turning. The descent.

I will never forget the moment of quickening with Connie. She was thirteen or fourteen weeks old. I was bundled up in this monster sweater that hung down to my knees. Lacey Woods had brought it back from somewhere in Central America, and it had this vaguely Aztec eagle on the back. It was beautiful, and so heavy that it kept me warm even outside on the sort of cold December day on which Connie made herself known.

I was sitting on one of the tremendous rocks in Mom and Dad's backyard, one of the ones that faced the ski resort on Mount Republic. Rand and I had decided by then we were going to get married, but the little one inside me wasn't the reason. She—of course, then it was still he or she, we hadn't a clue whether we'd be blessed with a boy or a girl—was just the signal that we might as well do it sooner rather than later.

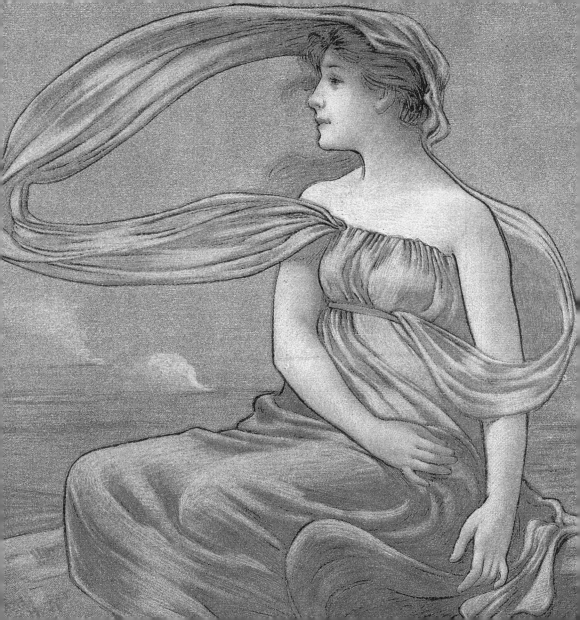

Midwives

The sun was already behind Republic, even though it wasn't quite four o'clock yet, and it was getting really chilly. They'd made some snow on the trails at the ski resort, but otherwise the ground was still brown, and so the mountain looked a little bit like a volcano that made this weird white lava.

I hadn't climbed those rocks since I was in high school, and sitting there made me feel like a very little girl. And then, suddenly, I felt this tiny flutter a bit below my belly button. A tadpole flicking its tail. A ripple, a wave. Instantly that image of the tadpole—an image I'd probably pulled from some high-school biology textbook—changed to that of a newborn baby. I knew my baby at that moment looked nothing at all like a newborn, but that was what I pretended was fluttering inside me. A psychedelic little person doing the breaststroke in a lava lamp. A bubble bouncing euphorically, but in slow motion, around in my tummy. I saw a newborn's pudgy fingers flicking amniotic fluid with a whoosh, I saw little feet smaller than baking potatoes gently splashing my own water against me, and I wrapped my arms around me and hugged my baby through my belly.

Midwives

Oh my God, was I happy. I remember I just sat on that rock grooving on the little person—my little person—inside me. Of all the little miracles that build to that big one, the birth itself, my favorite must be the moment of quickening. All these emotions and expectations and dreams for your baby just roll over you like so much surf.

And *quickening* really is the perfect word to describe it, because your heart races, and the pace of the pregnancy just takes off.

Some mothers experience the quickening as early as twelve weeks, others are much further along. Sixteen weeks is common in my experience, but some women don't feel it until they're through a good eighteen weeks. It really doesn't matter, except that those women who have to wait have to worry. It's inevitable, a mother can't help it. You want to feel your friend, you want to know he or she's there.

Of course, there may be one nice thing that comes with a later quickening. After all that anxiety, the high must be amazing when it finally arrives. Absolutely, unbelievably, outrageously amazing.

—*from the notebooks of Sibyl Danforth, midwife*

Bad heartburn? Well, the good news is your baby will be born with a full head of gorgeous hair! Or at least that's what the Old Wives say. While more reliable sources may disagree with the Wives' hairy predictions, all concur that, second only to morning sickness, heartburn is a leading pregnancy complaint.

Heartburn is a burning sensation occurring in the throat and chest area, from the bottom of the breastbone to the lower throat. Pregnant women may experience heartburn at any time of the day, though it often comes on within 30 minutes of eating or at night. Symptoms may be triggered by specific foods or by overeating, exercise, bending, or lying down.

Home Remedies:
Heartburn

Chances are, if you're suffering from heartburn, you already know it. But for an interesting test, stick out your tongue. According to traditional Chinese medicine, the tip of your tongue represents your heart. With heartburn, it is often tinged red. The middle of your tongue represents your stomach and digestive system, and it too may be very red.

So why heartburn? Your body is obviously going through great hormonal and physical changes. Traditional Chinese medicine says heartburn is linked to excessive heat in the stomach. Western medicine offers a similar theory: Hormones released during pregnancy can slow digestion and cause the valve between your stomach and esophagus to relax. Stomach acids can then seep up into your throat, causing that burning sensation. Also, as your baby grows, your uterus takes up more space, leaving less room for your stomach. Excess stomach acids have little place else to go but up!

Though there's no sure-fire heartburn preventive, here are some basic tips that might help you deter and ease your fiery symptoms:*

Avoid

- Rich, spicy, acidic, fatty, fried, and greasy foods.
- Foods containing chili powder and black, red, and hot pepper.
- Chocolate, peppermint, and spearmint.
- Oranges, grapefruit, and other acidic fruits and juices.
- Regular and decaffeinated tea and coffee, alcohol, and colas.
- Your personal trigger foods. For example—fresh bread, pastry, onions, red meat, cheese, or tomatoes.
- Overeating.
- Exercising immediately after eating.
- Bending over or lying down for at least two hours after meals.

Do

- Eat smaller meals 5–6 times a day.
- Eat slowly and chew thoroughly.
- Take a leisurely walk after meals.
- Drink smaller amounts of fluids more frequently.
- Sleep with your head elevated at least 6 inches (try adding extra pillows), or sleep upright in a comfy chair.

Try

- Eating a papaya for breakfast until symptoms improve.
- Chewing caraway, fennel, and dill seeds.
- A tablespoon of honey in a glass of warm milk.
- Drinking semi-skim milk to neutralize stomach acid.
- Fennel tea.

And if all else fails, see your caregiver—severe, continuous heartburn is a health issue that needs to be resolved.

*Always consult with your caregiver before taking antacids or natural supplements.

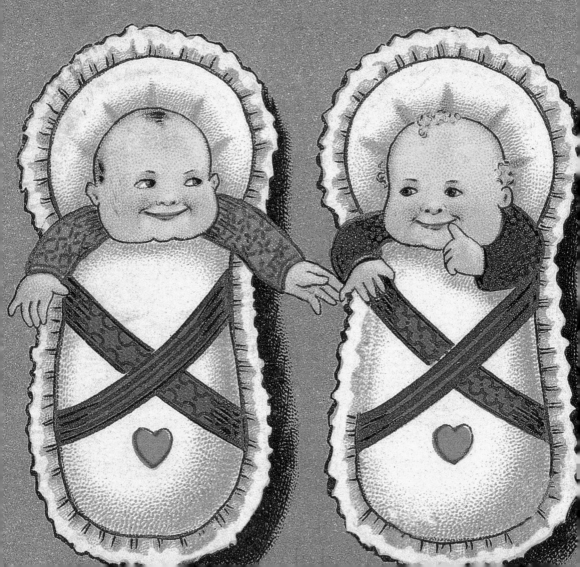

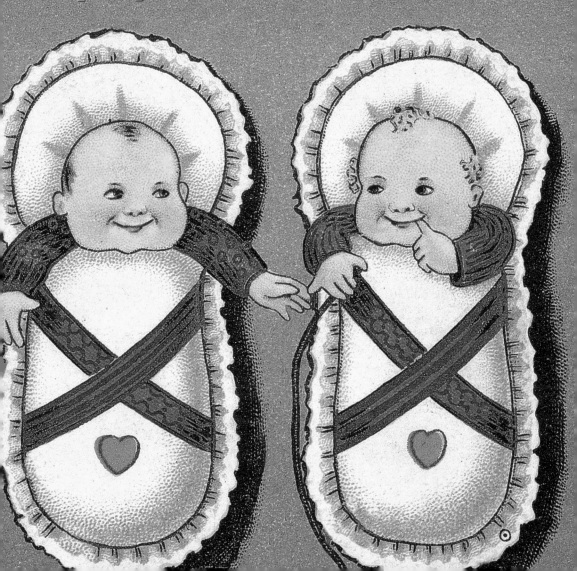

tart people.—*Don Herold*

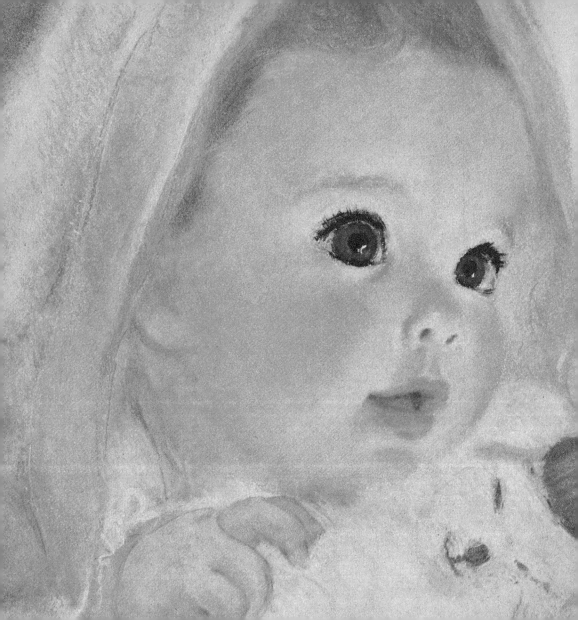

Life Within Life

Naomi Wolf

AT FOUR AND A QUARTER MONTHS I am due for a sonogram.
I appear at the medical building that sprawls over a part of Virginia
that only recently, my cabdriver tells me, was all apple orchards
and dairy farms. Passed from one smiling white-coated woman to
the next, I end up stripped to a gown, and lying under the cold
hands of a technician. There are no windows anywhere. The
technician, at once pert and professional, wipes a chilly gelatinous
substance on my belly.

I am alone, and filled with trepidation at who or what I will
encounter on the screen.

The technician moves the sensor over my abdomen like a
computer mouse. It feels odd to be, oneself, the informational field.
On the black-and-white screen tumble gray-blue clouds, like the
clouds of creation.

An oval emerges at length out of the chaos. "There you can see
the top of the fetus's skull," the technician says without inflection.
This is, after all, a routine part of her day, though to me it is the
introduction of a lifetime. My heart starts to race.

Life Within Life

She moves the mouse mysteriously over my abdomen, guided by some data that is unclear to me. "There you can see the back of its skull. Perfect," she remarks as colored digits and a measuring graph superimpose themselves over the image of this tiny chalice, the magic habitation of this creature's sensibility. "Right on track— just as big as it should be."

The skull vanishes, lost in the fog. "See that string of pearls?" she asks in her practiced voice. I squint at the screen. Out of the formlessness appears a sinuous x-ray serpent. It could be a strand of pearls, but the pearls of a fairy tale: a living, luminous thread. It shoots, undulating, through the darkness. I cannot recall ever seeing anything so beautiful. "See, each vertebra is there. Again, no visible defect."

Now the creature assembles itself against the mouse, manifesting its parts virtually with a will, as if it is battering against the membrane between us to make itself known to me. A hand appears, a forearm. The fist is utterly relaxed. There is nothing to grasp at yet. A foot, a footprint, white against the blackness; thin, ghostly shank, clumsy toes.

As I see that hand and that foot, something irrational happens; a lifetime's orientation toward women's rights over fetal rights lurches out of kilter. Some voice from the most primitive core of my

Life Within Life

brain—the voice of the species?—says: You must protect that little hand at all costs; no harm can come to it or its owner. That little human signature is now more important than you are.

The technician presses harder into what I would have guessed was some vital organ of mine; the creature—annoyed? playing?—shoots away from the sensor. We lose sight of it. "It's turning over," she says. "Somersaulting." Then we find it again.

I scarcely breathe. Now it is reclining on its back, practically resting on its elbows, knees bent, in profile, like the stone gods in Mexico. Its face is in profile too, a perfect, eerie, conventional snub-nosed baby profile.

Then slowly, as if it is looking straight at me—as if to warn me not ever, ever to take for granted its familiarity—it turns its face forward. The sweet baby profile dissolves and reconfigures itself. The down all over my skin rises.

The eyes are not human eyes, but the overscale almond eye-shields that have characterized images of malevolent space invaders for forty years. The vast, sightless eyes, the flat skull-nose and delicate nostrils, the bulging brow, the thin cruel line of the mouth—this is the face; this is where the mythology about aliens must come from. And in a way it is not surprising. Now that we've lit up the dark regions of the world with electricity, the fairies have

Life Within Life

fled. In Malaysia, they say that the ghosts vanished after the electric lights came on. What place is left for us to populate with alien beings except the dimensions of the womb?

"Do all four-month fetuses look like E. T.?" I ask the technician in a voice that tries for lightness. I will have to love this child whether it comes out looking like E. T. or not.

She laughs. "Oh, sure. I should have told you ahead of time. They all look like that. We get so used to it we forget to mention it—but parents are often spooked when they see the face for the first time."

Wiped off, and dressed in my street clothes, I hail a cab. I leave the building holding a full-color printout of my baby, the photo taken in its reassuring baby profile. This must be the convention for these images—to hide the alien helmet discreetly from the camera's eye. The technician presented it to me already framed in a cheap plastic cube, suitable for hanging on my kitchen wall. It looks like a souvenir from Disneyland. The fetuses all look like that, I comfort myself. But I can make only the weakest of efforts to remember this baby's face as more conventional, less "other."

Life Within Life

For, of course, it looks like an alien because it *is* an alien. Its true face is the one that turned the eyes of a whistling cosmos right at and through me. It is a baby in my belly but it is also a time-glider poised in inner space, ensouled already. Or to become ensouled, perhaps, at some moment that I will be unaware of, as I am steaming broccoli or reading the morning paper. Emergent from God alone knows where, suspended on its journey that I can never fathom, of course it is an alien; of course it looks like that.

I hang the picture on the nail in the kitchen that holds the Maurice Sendak calendar—"Alligators All Around" is the scene for July. But I look at it from time to time and know that, while this is the guise it will assume so I can love it and take it through life, its first face is older, stranger, and something derived form far beyond my species. "Oh, look at its nose!" exclaims Yasmin, my upstairs neighbor. "Sweet, sweet little hands, all cuddled up!" I look, and I will cherish that nose and those hands. But I am not fooled. And I could swear that, when it looked at me, it conveyed this directly: Yes, I will be a baby eventually: small, helpless, and humanly lovable. But not yet.

THE WOMB REPORT

🐛 It's my third week here in the womb, and I think I feel myself thinking. Hey, that must mean my brain is starting to develop!

Before I could feel only my mommy's heartbeat, but now there's a second one. It's small, like me. Wait—it's mine!

🐛 *5th week*: I was just floating around today, checking out my budding limbs. My eyes have started forming, but I won't be able to use them for a while. And there are these strange floppy things forming on the side of my head. I think I'll call them "ears," because that sounds funny…hee-hee…

Oh, and a nose has appeared on my face! I can't smell yet, but there's nothing much to smell around here anyway, except a whole lot of water. My arms look like flippers now, and my legs look like paddles, but I can't really move around. Maybe I'm becoming a fish….

🐛 *8th week*: Hey, I can move! It seems like my brain can control how my muscles move, and I've spent the day testing them out. Never too early to start exercising, you know. And you stretch to the left! Right! Left! Right!

Some handy-dandy fingers have formed on those flippers of mine in the last few days. I can bend my arms at the elbow too, which should help with my swimming. My cool tail is starting to get very stubby, and I think it might disappear soon.

3rd month: My mouth opens whenever anything touches my face. I can't help it—it's like a reflex. I have the beginnings of vocal cords now, too, but it's going to be a while before anyone can hear me crooning. I'm also practicing breathing and sucking with my muscles. Now that my arms are almost fully formed, I spend a lot of my time gliding through the sac. Soon I'll be able to flex my hands.

And my biggest news for the month: Teeth buds! Twenty of them! One day I'll be able to eat all sorts of yummy stuff.

4th month: I can kick now, but I don't think Mommy can feel me knocking around yet, because I only weigh in at about five ounces. I can feel my heart going *thumpity-thump* harder every day, and my eyes are now pointed straight ahead instead off to the side. I guess I'm not a fish, after all....

Inspired by my new taste buds, I've started making a list of things to try. So far I've got apple pie, hot dogs, corn syrup...

5th month: Last month I grew awfully fast, and it seems like this month will be no different. I'd guess I'm around 10 inches long now. Hmm, I wonder if Mommy can feel my kicks yet—I work hard to put every ounce of my one-pound self into each and every one. It's just my way of saying hi. Oh, and a light covering of soft hair has sprouted up all over my head and body! It's kind of neat, in a fuzzy-bear sort of way.

When I'm not busy spinning and somersaulting, I spend a good amount of time sleeping in my favorite position—with my chin resting on my chest.

6th month: This space is getting a little tight. I must be at least a foot long! Other than that, I don't have much fat yet, so my skin looks very wrinkly. Sometimes I can hear things too, like talking and music, outside the womb—and Mommy's stomach growling.

7th month: My eyelids have just opened for the first time. But there's not much to look at because it's so dark in here. Every now and then a little light glows through from outside Mommy's tummy and makes everything pink. I'm getting excited to see what the rest of the world looks like. On the other hand, it sure is warm and cozy in here....zzz...zzz...

8th month: Wow! Thumbs and fingers are really fun to suck on! But I've got to be careful not to scratch myself with my newly grown fingernails. My skin is becoming more smooth and opaque, and all five of my senses are ready to work! Plus, I've got a big brain to boot. I can tell that Mommy's getting excited about how fast I'm growing. Whenever I give her a loving kick in the belly, her heart beats really fast.

9th month: Wanna see me make a fist? I'm definitely getting stronger! I just passed the foot-and-a-half mark. I'm starting to get kind of chubby too, and it's making my elbows and knees dimple. It's becoming very difficult to move around in here, and most of the time I have to keep my arms crossed around my chest.

All right. Enough is enough! This big baby needs some more legroom. I think Mommy must agree, 'cause she sure is trying hard to push me out of here. You know, now that it's time, I'm having second thoughts about going. I mean, who knows what it's like out there? Maybe I'll hang on just a little longer....

Uh-oh, I'm losing my grip....

Wow! This is some ride!

Yippee! Look out world
—HERE COMES BABY!

Magnificat

Chana Bloch

1

Now the fingers and toes are
   formed,
the doctor says.
Nothing to worry about. Nothing
to worry about

2

I will carry my belly to the mountain!
I will bare it to the moon, let the
   wolves howl,
I will wear it forever.
I will hold it up every morning in
   my ten fingers,
crowing
to wake the world.

3

This flutter that comes with me
   everywhere
is it my fear

or is it your jointed fingers
is it your feet

4

You are growing yourself.
out of nothing:
there's nothing
at last I can
do: I stop
doing: you
are

5

Miles off in the dark,
my dark,
you head for dry land,

naked, safe
in salt waters.

Tides lap you.

Your breathing
makes me an ark.

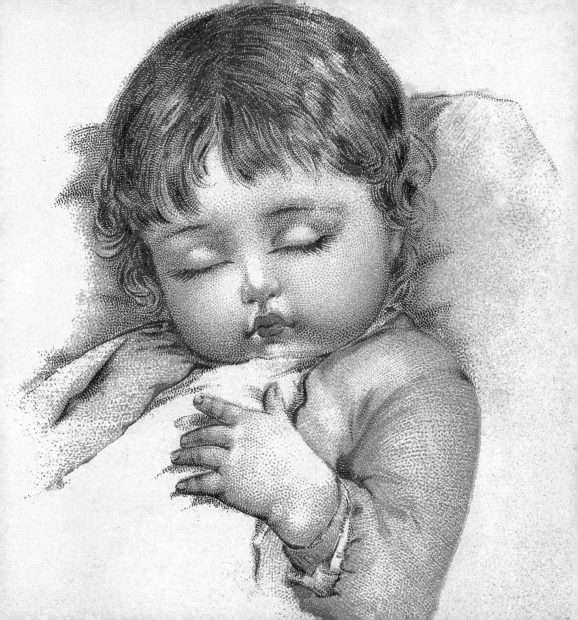

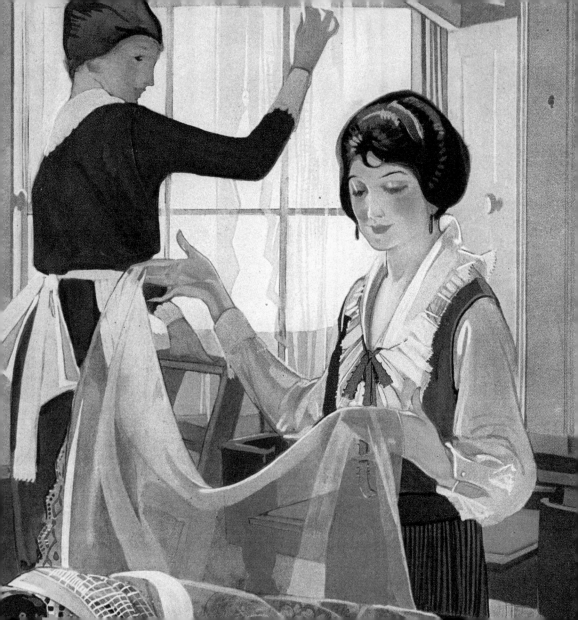

Special Tips

Decorating the nursery is a great way to personally welcome your child into his new home and satisfy those irresistible maternal nesting urges all at once. You want baby's room to be the most nurturing and beautiful haven possible. This is the space where your little one will spend most of his early days sleeping, eating, and observing his world. There are so many ways to make the nursery a special, soothing, and stimulating environment. Here are just a few ideas to inspire you.

A Crib with a View

Remember, your baby will sleep through much of her early life. That means she'll spend many hours in her crib examining the ceiling above. So give her something to look at! Hang mobiles or shiny crystals and paint pictures on the ceiling. Place the crib in the center of the room and give baby a panoramic view. Nothing delights an infant more than seeing her reflection. Secure a mirror to a wall near the crib and watch baby amuse herself for hours.

Sound Ideas

Sound is very important in the nursery. The music you listened to while you were expecting can comfort a cranky infant. The soft soothing trickle of a small water fountain or the tinkling of wind chimes also can relax baby (and mother, too.)

Clever Changing Table

Convert the top of a desk or chest of drawers into a changing table by adding a simple 3- to 4-inch-thick foam mat. Cut the foam 8 inches narrower than the desktop or chest. Trim a nonskid rug pad to the same size as the foam. Glue the pad to the bottom of the foam. Cover the top of the foam with waterproof sheeting. Wrap the top and sides of the foam neatly with a baby bath towel, which can be changed often. Presto! You've got a brand-new changing table!

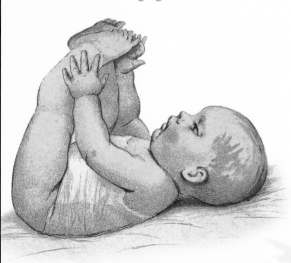

Antique Baby Dresser

An old armoire makes a great baby dresser. Add a fresh coat of white paint and install two closet rods (available at your local hardware store) in the top cupboard for hanging little clothes. Stack diapers on the bottom shelf.

Darling Details

After the basics (crib, drawers, rocker and pillow, lamp) indulge in details and follow a theme. Noah's Ark or a barnyard or zoo scene works well for an animal-loving family. Stencil an animal border, paint animal footprints on the floor, or hang stuffed-animal birds from the ceiling! Consider a nature motif with clouds on the ceiling, a butterfly mobile, and a painted family tree on the wall (see following pages for nature theme how-to.) Another unique idea: Frame your favorite children's book illustrations or paste them to the wall to make a very special border.

Nifty Thrifties

You don't have to spend a lot to be creative. Loads of decorative ideas can be implemented using what you already have. When seeking inspiration: Recycle! Save the ribbons from shower gifts to make a bright mobile, and the wrapping paper to line baby's drawers and shelves. Or make a collage on baby's closet door using all of the congratulatory messages and gift cards you've received, and shower invitations and birth announcements you've sent out.

Precious Laundry Bag

A simple and sweet laundry bag can be made with an "orphan" vintage pillowcase. Simply make two small holes in the hem of the case on either side of the seam. Attach a large safety pin to the end of one yard of 1-inch-wide grosgrain ribbon. Use the pin to manipulate the ribbon in one hole, through the hem, and out the other hole, creating a drawstring. Tie the ends of the ribbon together and hang the decorative bag on a doorknob or use to line a plastic pail for baby's laundry.

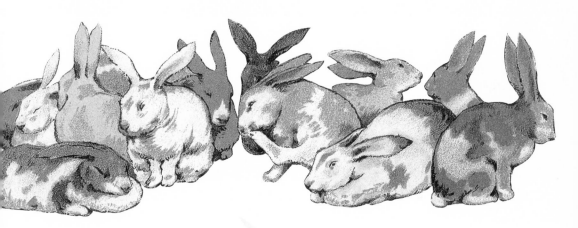

Sky Ceiling

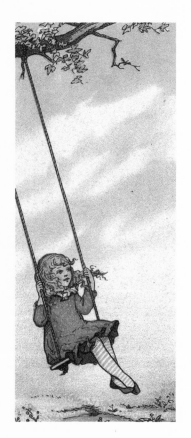

Bring the outside world inside your baby's nursery with a hand-painted sky ceiling. Recreate the comforting feeling of a warm spring afternoon as the clouds roll lazily overhead. It's easy to do, even if you're not particularly crafty! This view from the crib is certain to delight baby for years. As an added effect, decorate the ceiling with glow-in-the-dark stars and watch your nursery go from daytime to nighttime with a flick of a switch. This is also a neat decorating idea for a child's playroom.

You will need:

Latex interior wall paint in your favorite light blue
(I gal. = 350–400 sq. ft. per coat)

I pint white latex interior wall paint

Large paintbrush or roller and tray

I or 2 large natural sea sponges, slightly damp

Optional: acrylic craft/artists' paint

1. Prepare the ceiling as directed on the paint can and apply one to two coats (as necessary) of light blue paint. You may want to create a vaulted ceiling effect by extending the color down the walls several inches, making a border. Allow paint to fully dry after each coat.

2. Pour a little of the white paint into a disposable pie tin or plastic plate. Thin with an equal amount of water, adding a little at a time, mixing well.

3. To create clouds, lightly dip the damp sponge into the watered-down paint. Start from the center of each cloud and work outward in circles, repeatedly dabbing the sponge to apply an almost transparent white layer of paint in cloud shapes. Be creative. Vary the sizes and shapes of your clouds.

4. When you finish the first cloud layer, let it dry, and then sponge each cloud lightly again with a mixture of paint and half the amount of water, *allowing patches of the first layer to show through*, especially around the edges of your clouds.

5. Apply a third layer sparingly, highlighting your clouds with white undiluted paint, again allowing the first two layers to show through here and there.

6. If you're feeling especially creative, add a few passing birds or butterflies using the acrylic craft/artists' paint.

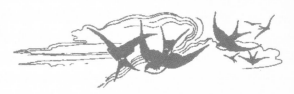

Homemade Mobiles

A mobile is a wonderfully entertaining part of baby's crib or bassinette. Infants are fascinated with light, blocks of color, shapes, and movement. You can make mobiles from just about any lightweight item that is baby-safe, just in case little hands grab ahold. Cut out animal pictures, angels, fish, flowers, or other shapes traced around your favorite cookie cutters, or use small stuffed animals. A mobile of family photos has special meaning and helps introduce baby to friendly faces. Or make a mobile for over the tub out of bright sponge cutouts from the craft store—it will have baby looking up when it's shampoo time! Here are two of our favorite mobiles to get you started.

You will need:

- 1 large sheet colored matte board
- 2 wire pants hangers (with cardboard tubing)
- Florist tape
- 1 yard $1/2$-inch-wide ribbon in any color
- Rubber cement
- Metal ceiling hook

For Family Photo Mobile:

- 16 close-up photographs of family faces (4˝ x 6˝ or 5˝ x 7˝) cut into various shapes
- 2 yards $1/4$-inch-wide satin ribbon

For Butterfly Mobile:

- Fishing line or nylon thread
- Large sewing needle
- Craft paint
- 16 matte-board butterflies

Family Photo Mobile

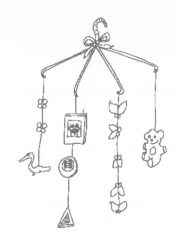

1. Select 16 close-up photos of the faces of family members, close friends, and even pets.

2. Cut matte board into 12 basic shapes— like circles, ovals, triangles, squares, diamonds, stars, hearts, and clouds— 3–5 inches wide.

3. Trim and glue photos of faces to the 16 matte-board shapes using rubber cement.

4. Remove the cardboard tubes from the wire hangers.

5. Hold the top "hooks" of the hangers together securely. Wrap tightly together with florist tape, including the twisted sections of the wires. Cover the tape by wrapping with ribbon. Tie a bow at the bottom of the taped hooks.

6. Bend the "wings" of the hangers at 90° angles so that they radiate in four directions.

7. Cut a 24-inch length of 1/4-inch ribbon.

8. Sandwich one end of ribbon between one cut-out photograph and the matching piece of matte board. Glue pieces together with ribbon lying flatly in between.

9. Leaving a few inches of ribbon in between each photograph, repeat step 2 two more times until you have three photo shapes glued to the ribbon at even intervals. Leave 3–5 inches of ribbon at the top to attach to mobile.

10. Repeat steps 7 through 9 three more times. Attach a piece of ribbon with photos to each of the four corners of the mobile.

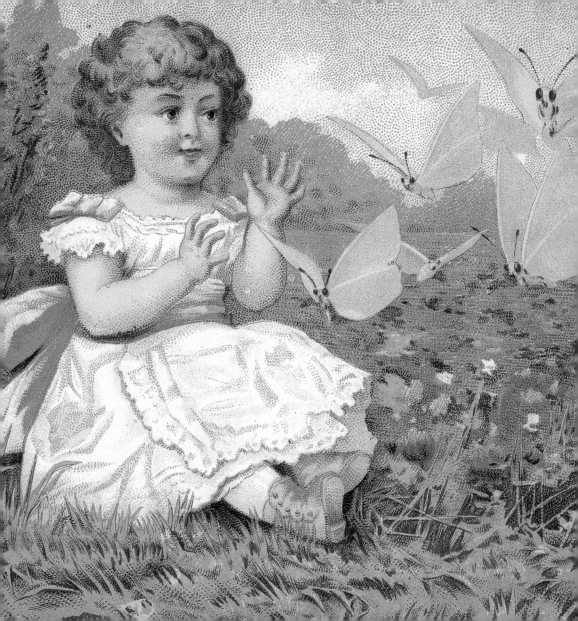

Butterfly Mobile

1. Cut matte board into 16 butterfly shapes 2 ¹/₂–4 inches wide and paint both sides in butterfly-wing designs; or paste on pictures, stickers, decals, or butterflies cut from gift paper.

2. Follow steps 4 through 6 of Family Photo Mobile.

3. Slightly bend each butterfly down its center. Set butterflies aside.

4. Cut a 15-inch piece of fishing line, tie a double knot at the end, and thread through the needle.

5. Pierce the underside center of a butterfly with the threaded needle and pull line through. Tie a knot several inches above the 1st butterfly and string a second butterfly onto the line. Repeat three more times, stringing three butterflies at different levels on each line. Repeat a fourth time, using an 18-inch piece of line and stringing four butterflies at different levels.

6. Hang one piece of 15-inch line from each of the four corners and the 18-inch piece of line from the center of the mobile. Attach lines by double-knotting around hanger wire. The mobile must have equal weight on all four opposing corners to hang evenly.

To Hang Mobile

1. Install ceiling hook above baby's crib by following the instructions on the back of the hook's packaging.

2. Take a length of fishing line and double-knot one end around the mobile's hook and the other end around the ceiling hook. Adjust length of line so that the mobile hangs above baby's reach. The finished mobile looks like a little swarm of butterflies or a crowd of friendly faces dancing above baby's bed.

Family Tree Mural

A family tree is a great way to encourage your new addition to learn about his ancestors and relatives. As a fixture in the nursery it helps baby become familiar with loved ones who live far away and generations to be remembered.

There are many ways to fashion a family tree, but a mural is easy and fun to make and provides a great decorative touch to baby's room. Created using potato stamp leaves, a bold painted trunk, and family photos, this is one tree that doesn't require a green thumb to bloom!

You will need:

Chalk

Craft paint

Small paintbrush

Tape measure

Straight-edge ruler

Family photos, scanned or copied and cropped to similar sizes

Wallpaper paste

Felt marker

Potato stamp in the shape of a leaf (*see following instructions*)

To Make Potato Stamp

1. Cut a large potato in two.

2. Carefully carve a leaf shape with a knife about ½ inch deep into the cut side of the potato, or press a leaf-shaped cookie cutter into the potato.

3. Cut away the potato flesh around the design so all that remains is a raised leaf shape.

To Make Family Tree Mural

1. Decide how many generations back your tree will go.

2. Measure the height you want your mural to be, and make a chalk mark at the top and bottom.

3. Divide the space into equal sections, marking one level for each generation.

4. Lightly sketch the tree. The trunk is for the names and photos of your children. Split the trunk into two branches (paternal side and maternal side). Draw two branches radiating upward from each of these (grandparents), then two more branches sprouting out and up from each of those (great-grandparents), and so on. You can add branches that extend horizontally, for aunts, uncles, and cousins.

5. Using brown craft paint thinned with water, paint in your trunk and branches.

6. Dip potato stamp in green craft paint and stamp leaves on the wall around all the branches.

7. Glue photos of family members to the appropriate branches with wallpaper paste. You can cut people out and have them standing, sitting, or dancing on the branches. Names and dates can be written either on the mural or on a chart that is framed and hung nearby.

8. Remember to add pictures to the mural each time your family grows.

Can I regard my pregnancy as
anything but one long festival?...
I especially remember how at odd
hours sleep overwhelmed me and
how I was seized again, as in my
infancy, by the need to sleep on the
ground, on the grass, on the sun-warmed
hay. A unique and healthy craving.

–Colette

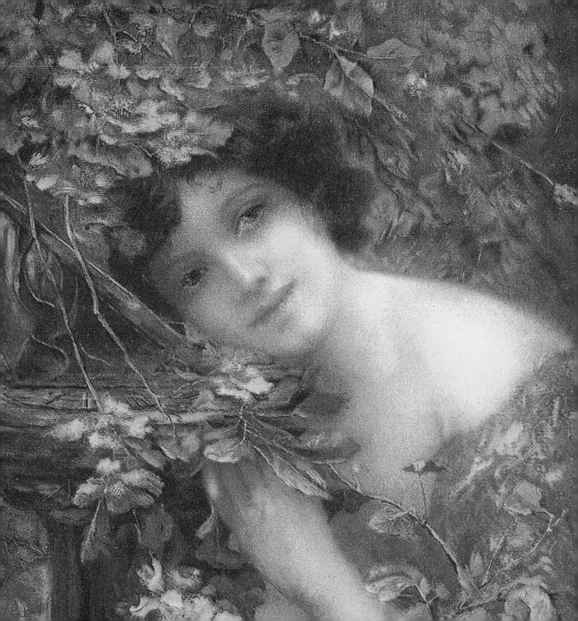

Peanut Butter and Lamb Chops

Paul Reiser

EVEN WITHOUT READING any "What to Expect" books, there are *some* things everyone knows to expect. You know, for example, from every old movie, TV show, joke, and established cliché that pregnant women are likely to crave peculiar foods and have unpredictable mood swings. But when you go through it yourself, you still can't believe what's going on.

One time, only a few weeks into pregnancy, I was awakened in the middle of the night to the sound of muted sniffling and the gentle smacking of pasty lips. Now, if it had been the lip-smacking *alone*, I would have assumed it was the dog, once again licking himself grotesquely and thoroughly. But the *sniffling* was new. The dog, while certainly a loving and sensitive animal, had never actually been moved to tears. I turned over to discover my wife sitting up and staring into space.

"You okay?"

"Mm-hmm."

"You sure?"

She said, "Ask me what I did from two-thirty to now."

"Okay. What?"

"Ate a banana and cried."

Peanut Butter and Lamb Chops

Okay. That was a sentence I had literally never heard. To my knowledge, eating a banana and crying is something you would do only if you were, say, auditioning for a part in a dramatic monkey movie.

I didn't know exactly what to say.

"Why are you crying?"

"I don't know."

"You want to talk?"

"No."

A few moments of silence.

"Do you want me to get you anything?"

"No, I'm so nauseous."

"How many bananas did you have?"

"Eight."

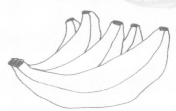

"Well," I thought to myself. "There you go. That might be part of the problem." But something told me it would have been woefully unproductive to say, "Honey, next time, maybe don't eat so many bananas at one time." Instead, I extended myself as lovingly and unconditionally as I knew how.

"Is there anything I can do for you?"

"Yeah—shut up and leave me alone."

This particular fun patch of your couplehood presents some of the juiciest, trickiest, and most explosive minefields that you will encounter in

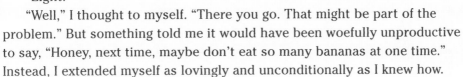

your linked-together little lives. Nowhere is a loving husband's ability to tap-dance, turn the other cheek, and "just walk away" put more relentlessly to the test.

The key to survival, I found, was in accepting that virtually nothing I did would be right. And if I *did* do something right, it was probably by accident. I reminded myself constantly that whatever horrific outbursts she unleashed, however vicious the attacks that came my way, they were all the result of tsunami-sized waves of surging hormones and should not reflect unnecessarily harshly on the Woman I Love. Until this phase blew over, I would just shake off these blows, pick myself up from the canvas, and again politely offer her my chin.

I think most husbands accept this pretty readily, because even the dumbest of the group knows that they're still getting off pretty easy. After all, it's not *their* bodies going through these violent upheavals.

I remember one night I felt my wife's head and was concerned she might be getting a fever.

"Gee, you seem hot," I said in an irrefutably sympathetic tone.

Her response?

"Yeah, maybe it's because I'm in @#*!#-ing *HELL*."

Apparently, that's not uncommon. When you're in @#*!#-ing hell, your forehead can feel a wee bit feverish. (By the way, that's the way my wife

Peanut Butter and Lamb Chops

actually curses. She doesn't use dirty words; she'll literally say "asterisk, pound sign, exclamation point, the-letter-'A'-with-a-circle-around-it, asterisk, asterisk, asterisk.")

I thought I was prepared for the food cravings. Having seen enough *I Love Lucy* reruns growing up, I was all set to run out, any time of day or night, for pickles and ice cream. As it turns out, my wife had no interest in either pickles *or* ice cream. However, we couldn't get our hands on enough peanut butter and lamb chops. Peanut butter and lamb chops—which was also, interestingly enough, the name of a delightful children's show I enjoyed as a young boy—were not foods that had ever been a significant part of our life before pregnancy. In fact, my wife almost never ate *either*.

So where did these cravings come from? I concluded it's the baby, *ordering in*. Prenatal takeout. Even without ever being in a restaurant, fetuses develop remarkably discerning palates, and they are not shy about demanding what they want. If they get a hankering, they just pick up that umbilical cord and call.

"You know what would taste good right now? A cheeseburger, large fries, and a vanilla shake. And if you could, hurry it up, because I'm supposed to grow lungs in a half hour."

CRAZY CRAVINGS

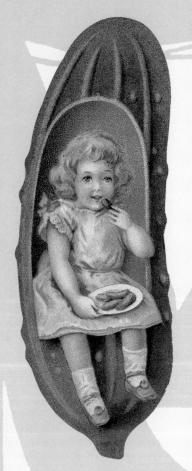

Are you constantly running to the store for more chocolate mint ice cream? Is your appetite for greasy fries impossible to curb? Well, you're not alone. Statistically speaking, more than two-thirds of all women report at least one strong food craving during pregnancy. Shifting hormones, an altered sense of taste and smell, and changes in your nutritional requirements are to blame. Some women have an insatiable desire for sweets, particularly chocolate. Others crave salty foods, like olives, pickles, and potato chips. But are all cravings bad?

Most healthcare professionals agree that a yearning for a particular food is only bad insomuch as it causes an imbalance in your diet. So, try to satisfy your yens with a variety of foods, and avoid the junk-food cravings by finding substitutes. Next time the salt bug bites, pass on the bottomless bag of fatty potato chips. Reach instead for baked chips or soft pretzels. Satisfy your passion for a hot-fudge sundae or chocolate shake with a nonfat frozen yoghurt or smoothie. And if you crave oranges, nectarines, broccoli, and collard greens, consider yourself lucky and, by all means, indulge!

THE PROVERBIAL PICKLES AND ICE CREAM

Bizarre culinary combinations abound during pregnancy. And, although we don't know any mothers who'd kill for pickles dipped in Rocky Road, here's what some had to say about their cravings:

"During my first trimester, I craved the foods of my childhood. When I was little my mom would make grilled-cheese sandwiches and tomato soup, tuna melts, cottage cheese and fruit (in sweet syrup, of course), and macaroni and cheese with hot dogs—very glamorous foods, all. But that wasn't even the worst of it. My cravings for the sweets of my youth also returned in full force. Try reigning in an obsession for Necco wafers, Sweet Tarts, and Red Vines. I'm just lucky that Fun Dip is so hard to find these days."

"When I was pregnant with my daughter, I longed for mushrooms. This fact astonished me, as I had never been a mushroom enthusiast—in truth, I was quite the opposite. Sure enough, as soon as she was born, my aversion returned."

"With each of my pregnancies, I have experienced an overwhelming desire for anything orange—carrots, yams, and sweet potatoes; peaches, papaya, and cantaloupe; pumpkin pie, butterscotch pudding, and orange sherbet. And I can't leave out the goldfish crackers! If it was orange...I was eating it."

"Apples! That's all I wanted, for breakfast, lunch, and dinner."

So, the next time you wake up at two in the morning with a yen for yams and Jell-O, don't feel guilty. Just remember, it comes with the territory.

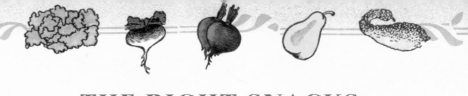

THE RIGHT SNACKS

Finding it harder to pack a full meal into your ever-shrinking stomach? Does your hunger strike more frequently these days? Try eating smaller meals more often. In truth, it is a healthier way to live—as long as you're making sound food choices. So, next time you have a snack attack, reach for something healthy. Bite down on a banana or whole-wheat crackers and some low-fat string cheese. Munch on an apple and some yoghurt, half a peanut butter and jelly (preferably whole-fruit spread) sandwich and a pear, edamame (green soy beans in the pod), low- or nonfat cottage cheese and fruit, dried fruits and nuts, or a bowl of cereal and milk. Or try one of our recipes.

HOMEMADE GRANOLA
(Benefits: This low-fat, low-sugar treat provides a lasting energy boost.)

Ingredients
1 ½ cups rolled oats
¼ cup chopped almonds
2 tablespoons sugar
1 ½ tablespoons ground cinnamon
Optional: dried cherries, cranberries, or apricots; raisins; wheat germ; and sunflower or pumpkin seeds.

1. Preheat oven to 350 degrees.

2. Combine all ingredients in a medium bowl and mix well. Spread the mixture on a baking sheet or in a shallow pan.

3. Bake for 25 to 30 minutes, or until light brown, stirring frequently. Let cool completely and then store in an airtight container. Granola should keep for at least a week.

4. Serve with fruit, yoghurt, or as a topping for ice cream or frozen yoghurt.

Makes 2 cups.

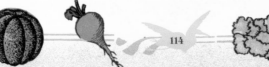

THE RIGHT SNACKS

LEMONY HUMMUS

(Benefits: Chickpeas are a terrific source of vitamin C; they contain more iron than any other legume, and aid in spleen, pancreas, stomach, and heart function. The garlic and lemon both help to cleanse the blood of toxins.)

Ingredients
1 clove garlic
4 teaspoons lemon juice
1 15-ounce can chickpeas
(garbanzo beans)
2 tablespoons tahini (sesame paste) or sesame seeds

1. Sauté garlic in 2 tablespoons lemon juice until soft.

2. Place all ingredients in blender and purée until smooth.

3. Serve in a whole-wheat pita pocket as a sandwich or as a dip with fresh vegetable pieces. Garnish dip with ground paprika, coarsely chopped parsley, and extra virgin olive oil.

Makes 2 cups.

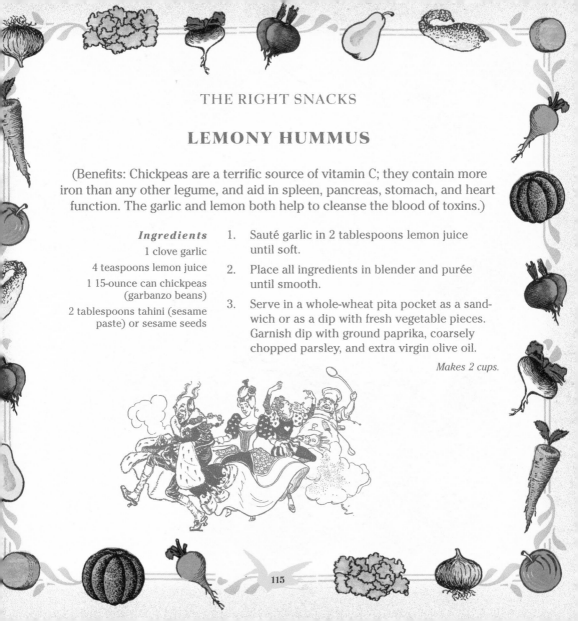

SIMPLE QUESADILLA

(Benefits: With the right fillings, this tasty
snack doubles as a well-balanced mini-meal.)

Ingredients

1 ounce reduced-fat cheddar or
Monterey Jack cheese

2 whole-wheat or
spinach tortillas

Optional: low-fat canned refried
beans, chopped tomatoes,
leftover chicken or shrimp,
sautéed onions, fresh spinach,
sautéed chopped bell peppers,
minced garlic, whole pinto
beans, salsa, chopped oregano,
chopped cilantro, low- or nonfat
sour cream, leftover rice,
slices of avocado and olives.

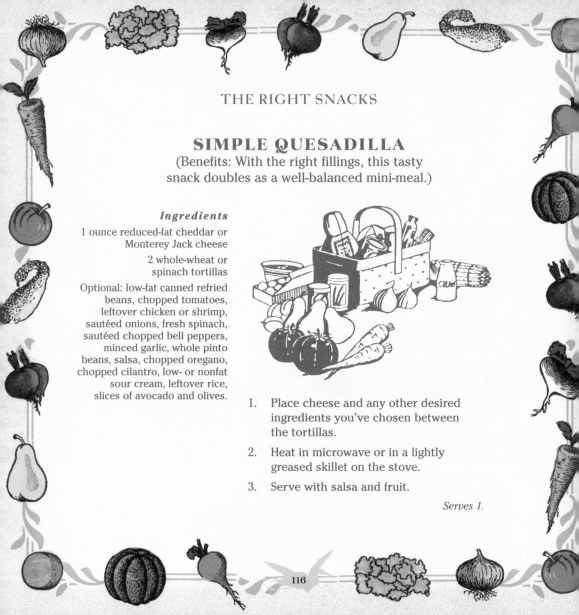

1. Place cheese and any other desired
   ingredients you've chosen between
   the tortillas.

2. Heat in microwave or in a lightly
   greased skillet on the stove.

3. Serve with salsa and fruit.

Serves 1.

FRUITY SOY POPSICLES

(Benefits: Mangoes are a good source of vitamin A and niacin—both
essential aids to your baby's growth and development. Soymilk is an
excellent source of protein, B-vitamins, and iron. Look for brands that are
fortified with calcium and vitamin D. Note: Vary this recipe by substituting berries, bananas, or other fruits for the mangoes; avoid choosing
citrus, however, as it may cause the soymilk to curdle.)

Ingredients
2 medium-size mangoes
2 cups soymilk
$\frac{1}{2}$ teaspoon vanilla extract

1. Peel mangoes and slice fruit away
    from seeds.

2. Purée ingredients in blender until
    smooth. (Optional: Reserve half the
    mango to blend in briefly at the end,
    so fruit chunks remain in the mixture.)

3. Pour mixture into ice-cube trays.
    Place in the freezer for 3–5 hours to
    harden. Add toothpicks or half
    Popsicle sticks after one hour.

Yields 2 ice trays.

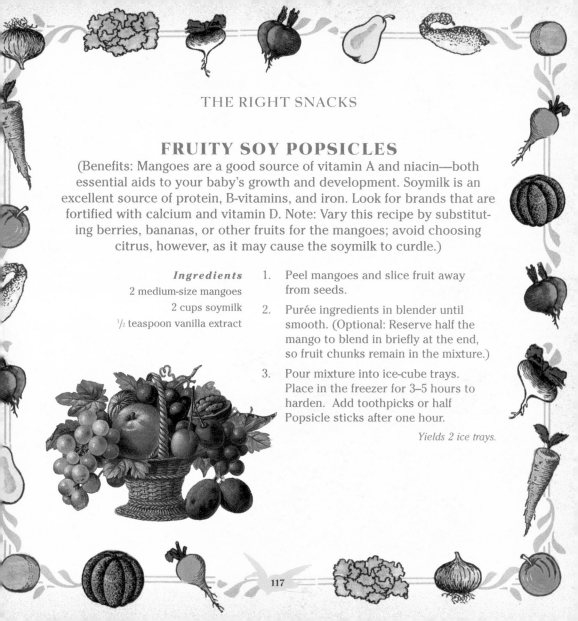

Madame Bovary

Gustave Flaubert

Translated by Francis Steegmuller

HE HAD another, happier concern—his wife's pregnancy. As her term drew near she became ever dearer to him. Another bond of the flesh was being forged between them, one which gave him an all-pervasive feeling that their union was now closer. The indolence of her gait, the gentle sway of her uncorseted body, her tired way of sitting in a chair, all filled him with uncontrollable happiness: he would go up to her and kiss her, stroke her face, call her "little mother," try to dance with her; and half laughing, half weeping, he would think of a thousand playful endearments to shower her with. The idea of having begotten a child enchanted him. Now he had everything he could ever hope for. He had been granted all that human life had to offer, and he was serenely ready to enjoy it.

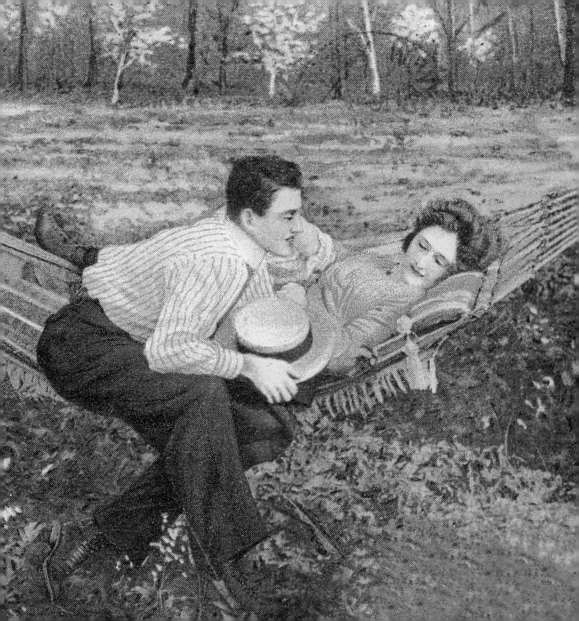

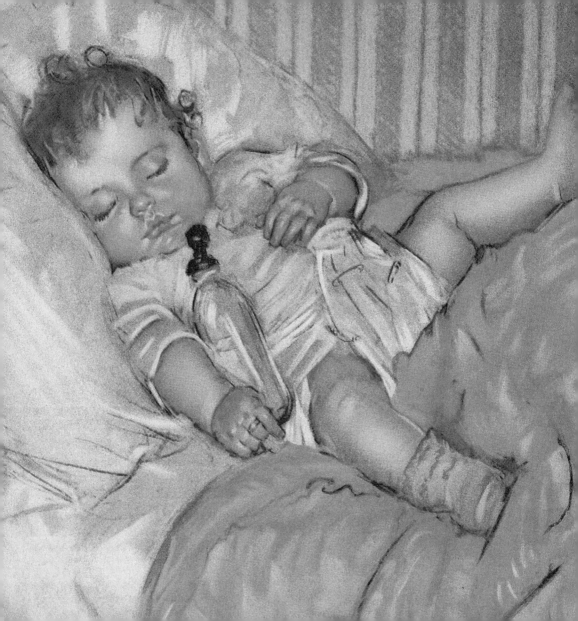

Postcard to My Unborn Son

Kirk Robertson

I just thought
since you're all curled
up inside there
I'd tell you about it
how it was
when your mother and I
came together

In a moon of cherries
Squirrel ran up a tree
Wind blew but stopped
when the pipe was lit
the breath trapped
in small buckskin pouches

I was told *you will*
have a tough life
all you can do
is go through it

That's how small things
survive like grass
pushing up through
cracks in the asphalt

Husbands Have Fears
of Their Own

Vicki Iovine

NOT THAT I AM SUGGESTING that it is your job to do anything about it, but it might be nice to occasionally remind yourself that you are not the only one who is turning into a parent in the foreseeable future. You are not the only one in your house with worries and concerns. Husbands have fears of their own, and what follows is a list of most of them, in no particular order:

1. If He Becomes a Father, He Cannot Be the Baby Anymore.

A lot of us are married to men who require a certain amount of mothering to keep them happy. They like being nurtured and coddled, and they worry, with good reason, that you will have less time to do this for them if you are doing it for the baby. As my husband so succinctly put, "You are like a pie. Every time you get pregnant, my piece of the pie gets smaller."

2. A Baby Is So Expensive That the Family Will Go Broke.

Even if you don't go bankrupt immediately, at the very least your husband won't be able to get that jukebox he has always wanted. This money worry is often at the top of the charts for husbands, probably because they are

Husbands Have Fears of Their Own

traditionally expected to provide for the baby, at least while you are incapacitated, and they don't know if they are up to the job. Even if you are a two-income family and you intend to return to work shortly after delivering, the truth remains, babies *are* expensive, and they only get more expensive as they get older. Most of us, however, have already decided that the financial sacrifices are worth it, or else we wouldn't have gotten pregnant in the first place.

3. His Wife Will Get Ugly.

Well, maybe that is stated too harshly. Perhaps it is more accurate to suggest that he is just afraid of not feeling as sexually aroused by the new and enlarged version of his wife. Or maybe he pictures women who don't get out of their bathrobes or wash their hair often enough when they get pregnant, and he worries that you will be like them.

4. His Wife Will Never Go Back to Her Old Self.

Remember, your husband fell in love with a woman who looked a certain way, and pregnancy is most certainly going to change that look dramatically. Even those men who think that their pregnant wives are sexy, or cute, occasionally have to wonder whether they will do what it takes to get their old figures back, more or less, or if they will be forever altered. Look at Grace Kelly, Elizabeth Taylor or other such former beauties. They never again looked like they did in *Father of the Bride* or *Rear Window* after having birthed a few children. (We should all look so bad, right?) So, it can clearly happen to the best of us.

5. The Rational, Stable Wife He Used to Have Will Be Permanently Replaced by This Sobbing, Sleepy, Impatient, Ravenous, Baby-Obsessed Person Who Has Gas.

No matter how much he wants to believe that this whole matter of pregnancy-induced insanity is a temporary state of affairs, he will worry that the old, fun you will never come back. It is so hard for men to imagine the emotional effect pregnancy has on a woman, never having experienced pregnancy or even PMS themselves, that they secretly suspect that this moodiness is not simply baby-related, but clear evidence of psychosis. If their friends with kids have told them anything about postpartum depression, then they worry that you will continue to be crazy even after the baby is born.

6. He Will Panic When His Wife Goes Into Labor and Be Unable to Find His Way to the Hospital.

Just as we have nightmares in which we misplace our babies, husbands have all sorts of nightmares about how they will mess up at the Big

Husbands Have Fears of Their Own

Moment. Every time they drive you to the hospital, whether for a tour, Lamaze classes or because you are making them practice, they will imagine trying to make the drive when their brains are rendered useless by terror. But don't *you* worry about your husband forgetting how to get to the hospital, because *you* will remember, and you will be yelling directions at him the whole way.

7. He Will Have to Deliver the Baby Himself.

He imagines the car breaking down or a blizzard or some other disaster occurring at the moment you most need to get to a hospital, and single-handedly having to deliver the baby. That fear is not totally outside the realm of rationality, because nearly all of us have heard at least one story of a couple's encountering a hazard that almost prevented them from getting to the hospital. My brother-in-law was backing the car out of the garage during a January snowstorm in New York to take my sister-in-law to the hospital to have her baby. He had the driver's door open so that he could see clearly as he reversed down the slippery driveway. The door caught on a snowdrift and ripped right off the car. Do you think that stopped them from getting to the hospital on time? Not on your life. People are capable of amazing feats when they panic, and driving with no door was not going to get in the way of this delivery occurring in a professional setting.

Husbands Have Fears of Their Own

8. He Will Faint During Delivery (or Worse Yet, He Will Stay Conscious and Have to Watch the Whole Thing).

I think most men imagine fainting in the delivery room because it is one of those clichés from television and movies. Labor and delivery are not rapid, catch-you-off-guard occurrences, but rather slow and deliberate progressions. Therefore, they are not the kinds of things that make people faint. Vomit, perhaps, but not faint.

9. The Doctor Will Insist That He Cut the Umbilical Cord.

Now this, on the other hand, does have some fainting elements to it. For one thing, the cord looks unquestionably like a part of the human biology, and therefore not like something that most people are inclined to want to damage in any way. Second, when you cut it, *stuff*, like blood, can come squirting out. If he doesn't know that in advance, your husband just may have his fainting fear come true. My Girlfriend Dona absolutely forbade her husband to cut her daughter's umbilical cord. Given his mechanical ability, it didn't seem like a very good idea. It wasn't all that high on his wish list, either, so he was only to happy to leave the task to professionals.

10. Labor and Delivery Will Hurt His Wife, and He Won't Be Able to Make It Better.

This is a very common and very sweet concern among husbands. Most of my Girlfriends have told me that the hardest part of having a baby for their husbands was having to watch the women they love suffer. They don't know what to do to make it better, and they may feel faintly guilty at the passive role they must play. (And if they don't, most laboring wives will see to it that they do.) My own husband used to beg me to ask for an epidural the minute I changed out of my clothes and into a hospital gown. His thinking was, "We know this is going to hurt eventually, so do us both a favor and take the drugs now."

11. He Will Never Be Able to Have Sex With His Wife Again.

A substantial number of men like to think of breasts and vaginas as being designed for one thing: THEM. Intellectually, they know that these organs will have to be shared with the new baby, but sexually, they don't want to know about it. Many husbands have wondered if they would ever want to have intercourse with their wives again if they were to see a bowling ball come out of her down there. My Girlfriend Patti never discussed this possibility with her husband; she simply headed the whole thing off at the pass by forbidding him to stand anywhere but at her head during delivery. If her doctor were to have offered to move a mirror down there so that both of them could see the baby crowning, she would have risked the seven years' bad luck and broken it over his head.

12. His Wife Will Die and Leave Him With Some Strange Baby.

Both men and women admit to having irrational fears about the wife dying in childbirth; the wife is concerned for obvious reasons, and the husband fears that, in addition to losing someone he is rather fond of, he will be on his own with the baby. With rare exception, men think of tending to newborn babies as woman's work, and they have a hard time imagining doing all of the caring and nurturing involved in raising a child without the mother as the primary caretaker. Since this baby is still a stranger to him, and his wife is his family, he also worries that he would resent the baby if it were to hurt his wife in any way. By the way, because you are probably a mite sensitive at this time in your life, let me remind you of what you already know: It is almost unheard of in this day and age for women to die in childbirth.

13. He Is Bound to This Woman Forever.

When you are married without children, the thought of breaking up can be heartbreaking, but you figure you can make the split somehow and eventually get on with your lives. Once the two of you have children together, however, you are in each other's life in a very real way for decades, whether you want to be or not. They are a joint, ongoing project that you will have in common no matter who else you may fall in love with or how much un-in-love the two of you may someday grow to be. The good news is, children keep you so busy and distracted that you may not even notice if your marriage has gone to pot.

14. He Won't Be as Good a Father as His Father Was.

A good father is the stuff from which heroes are created. (A mother, no matter how good or bad, becomes the motivation for psychiatric therapy later in her children's lives.) If a man admired and loved his own father, there is sometimes the fear that he could never do the job as well himself. After all, *he* is merely a thirteen-year-old in a man's body, and *his father* was, well, a FATHER. The truth is, once he has a child of his own, your husband will come to see his father for the human being that he was, as uncertain about but as devoted to the job of child rearing as he himself is now.

15. He Will Be as Good a Father as His Father Was.

This is the real world, and a lot of men grew up with less-than-ideal fathers, or even with no fathers at all. If your husband was not all that enamored of his own father's parenting abilities, he may be intimidated about becoming a father himself. There are no books or classes that teach you how to parent properly. If you are lucky, you learn it though emulation of your own parents. That sometimes leaves the people with no role models pretty much up in the air. Or worse, they develop unrealistic expectations for parenthood based on their own childish fantasies of what a *good* daddy would have been like, fantasies that are themselves based on fairy tales and television sitcom fathers.

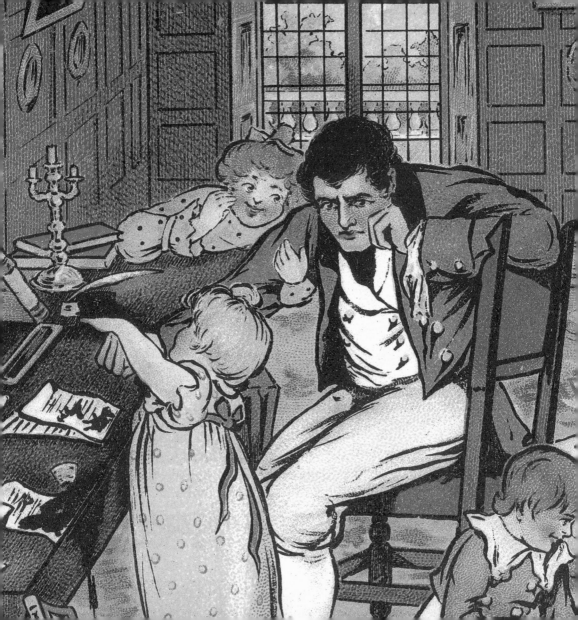

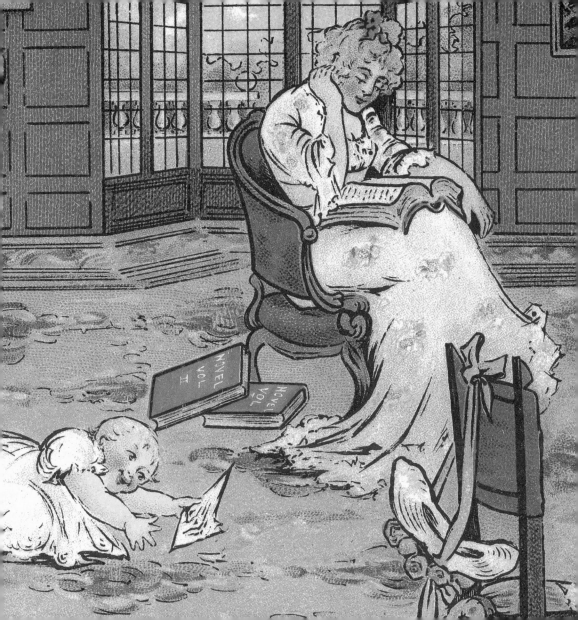

Having a child is surely the most beautifully irrational act that two people in love can commit.

–*Bill Cosby*

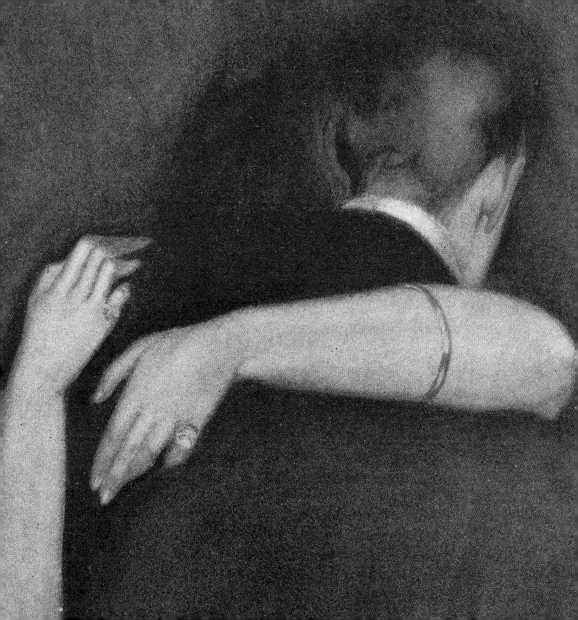

Mortal Terrors and Motherhood

Amy Herrick

I WILL SAY FIRST, I was not a girl carried away by a passion for babies. I didn't avoid them, but neither did they loom large in my ambitions.

When the King of My Mountain announced that he had set his heart on one, I was taken aback. We're too young, I said. We don't know what we're doing. What if we drop it? What if we ruin its character?

He brushed my fears aside with a wave of his hand. He said that we'd do as good a job as anybody else. More was not necessary.

I was nudged along on some current I could not name. I wanted to know who was the responsible party in such matters. Was it destiny? Were we just dupes of nature?

In the end I agreed to give it a try because I figured it might be one of those things I'd regret never having done, like eating sushi or riding the Cyclone at Coney Island. It wasn't that I exactly wanted to do it, but I was worried that if I didn't do it, I would always wonder what I'd missed.

Mortal Terrors and Motherhood

If this was not an ideal motive for bringing a new and innocent person into the world, still, I think it was the only one that could have carried me over the pass.

Several months later I peered down at the little blue line which had appeared on the home pregnancy test kit. Beneath the great thrill of absurd pride that I experienced at this accomplishment, I felt a cold shadow of fear slide by, silent and sharklike.

I went into the other room, where my husband was blithely reading the sports section and leaving coffee rings all over everything, and told him the news that he'd better get his act together, as things were about to change. Then I went into the kitchen to make myself breakfast, but found myself, again, gripped by a queasy chill of fear.

What was it? Was it the thought of the method by which this thing had gained entrance to my insides, or the thought of how it was—even now—wildly doubling and tripling in size by sucking up my juices through a cord attached to its bellybutton? Or was it the rather unbelievable idea of how it would eventually make its exit?

Mortal Terrors and Motherhood

I didn't know exactly, but who in their right minds would volunteer for such an experiment?

When the Other Party came in a little later and sat down nervously next to me and asked me what was the matter, I, naturally, could not really tell him. He patted me in that lame way guys pat you when they don't really want to know what's going on, and then, when that didn't seem to be sufficient, he put his arms around me. "What is it? Tell me."

"I'm afraid," I said at last, sobbing.

"Afraid? Afraid of what?"

"I don't know."

"But it's going to be great, really great. We can take it to the zoo and the museum. We'll have an excuse to buy Hawaiian Punch and you can put it in your lap and go down that twisty slide in the playground you always wanted to go down. We're gonna have a lot of fun. Really."

Of course, he was right. What was there to be afraid of? Zillions of people had babies. There was no reason I couldn't pull this thing off.

And for the next few days, although I was nagged by a sense of unease, there was nothing of any substance that I could put my finger on and I began to relax.

Mortal Terrors and Motherhood

Then, one afternoon, I went into the kitchen to have some tea and I happened to pick up one of my Everything You Need to Know About Being Pregnant handbooks and my eye just happened to fall on the section about Toxoplasmosis.

Toxoplasmosis is a disease you can get from handling cat poop and it's very sinister because the mother often has no symptoms or she thinks she's just got a cold, but meanwhile it slips across the placenta and causes the baby to go blind and deaf. When you're pregnant, the book said, it is wise to wear gloves when gardening in case you inadvertently brush up against any leavings of any stray cats.

Just an hour before I had been gardening and I had not been wearing gloves.

I was instantly plunged into a state of the most frantic despair and gloom, certain that I had contracted this hideous germ. I refrained, however, from mentioning what was on my mind to anybody, because part of me was pretty sure I was a lunatic.

After a couple of days, when my husband finally threatened to put his head in the oven if I didn't tell him what was wrong, I told him.

Being a wise man, he did not bother to get into an argument with me, but suggested I call our obstetrician (which was what I was dying to do, but hadn't been able to get up the nerve for) and talk to him about it.

Mortal Terrors and Motherhood

When I called my obstetrician, he suggested I go to the lab and get a blood test done.

The blood test came back negative. I was almost prostrated with relief.

On the other hand, all I could think about was what a terrible person I was, what a horrible mother I was going to make. What good mother would mind that her child was deaf and blind?

I wept with sorrow and relief and vowed to take the experience as a warning that if I was going to survive the next few months I must learn how to sit back and relax.

My water broke at around one in the morning. I had just fallen asleep when I felt this strange trickling sensation on my thighs. I stumbled bulkily out of bed and rushed to the bathroom. As I stood frozen with excitement on the tile floor, there was another small gush of water. The doctor had said check the color of the water to make sure the baby wasn't in distress. Clear water was good. Green water was bad. I caught a small splash in my hands and tried to examine it.

"Get me a cup!" I yelled.

"Whaddaya mean?" my husband yelled irritably. "I'm asleep! Get your own cup."

Mortal Terrors and Motherhood

"For crying out loud, I think my water just broke!"

In the next instant, my beloved teammate, who up to this point had seemed to take the prospect of becoming a father as casually as he would a shopping trip to buy socks, suddenly appeared in the doorway in a crouch, with a strange look on his face, as if he were a quarterback, as if he thought I was about to throw the baby to him.

"Did you get the cup?" I asked him.

He looked at me intently, as if I were speaking Portuguese. Then he spun around and disappeared. He returned a moment later with a clean coffee mug. I opened my palms and emptied the water into it.

We both stared down into the water as if our lives depended on it, as if we expected to see down there a map, a sign, a face. Something to tell us what our next move ought to be.

But all we saw was baby pee, a little funky smelling, but perfectly clear.

Several hours later, I lay in my hospital bed waiting for my newly arrived son, who was sleeping next to my bed in his little plastic bassinet, to wake up and have a feed.

As I lay there I was filled with a delicious anticipation. It was almost as if, in some confusion of identity with the little one who lay next to me, I was waiting for some exquisite food that I could not name.

Mortal Terrors and Motherhood

He had been sleepy and calm when he'd first arrived, not interested in eating, and I couldn't wait to see what nursing would be like.

I had had a little anxiety when, an hour earlier, they had brought him in to me from the nursery where they had been giving him his post-delivery clean-up. I had been afraid that I wouldn't recognize him, that I was not a good enough mother to recognize her own child. But as soon as they lowered him into my arms I was completely reassured. All was right with the world. I was home free. He was slimy and squish-faced, but he was perfect, and I knew that I could have picked him out of a crowd of ten thousand.

Now I lay there, waiting peacefully for my little one to wake up and have his first dinner. After an hour or so, he stirred and flexed his little hands and did not cry, but began to make tiny, comic little animal sounds. I lifted him carefully out of his bassinet and fumbled with the buttons of my gown and stuck my breast in his face.

For a brief minute, he opened his eyes and looked up at me with a frown as if he were wondering who the hell I was. Still frowning, he made a sleepy, completely uncoordinated attempt to get the nipple in his mouth and then he fell back asleep.

Mortal Terrors and Motherhood

I was filled with panic. Something was wrong. He hadn't nursed in the delivery room and he still didn't seem to be hungry. What could be going on?

Failure to thrive.

When the nurse came in I was weeping. "Something's wrong," I told her. "He won't suck."

She raised her eyebrows and, with a deft and casual hand, grabbed the baby and directed him to my nipple. With the other hand she gave my breast a quick squeeze. The baby opened his eyes very wide, bicycled his tiny legs in excitement, and with a ferocious lunge clamped down and began to drink like somebody who'd been lost in a desert for nine months.

He was fine. He was perfect.

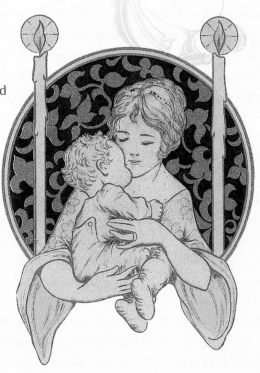

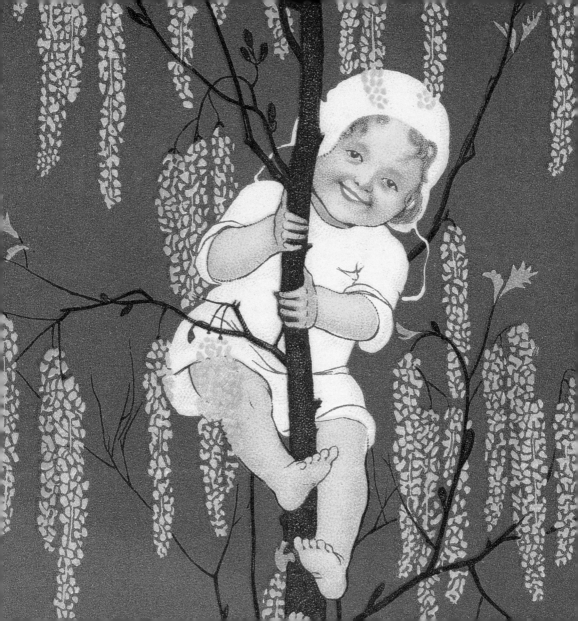

The rules for parents are
but three...Love, Limit,
and Let them be.

–Elaine M. Ward

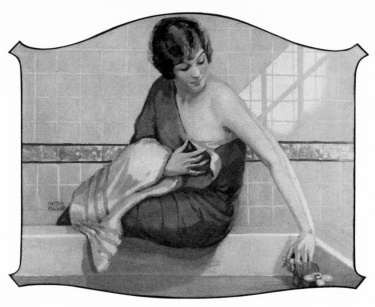

SPA DAY

Pregnancy can be a stressful time. You can even get stressed worrying about stress! Eating well, getting your rest, exercising, and stretching all help keep you balanced. But sometimes you need a little extra pampering. So, go ahead. Put your feet up. Walk in the fresh air. Read a book. Watch an old movie. Better yet, take a "spa day" for yourself, or at least a spa hour. Here are some suggestions:

Soothing Soaks

What could be better than slipping into a tub of warm water? A cozy bath can do wonders for lack of energy, sore muscles, insomnia, and the strain your increasing girth places on your body. And these are just the physical benefits!

1. Start by turning your bathroom into a sanctuary. Light some candles. Play restful music. Prop up your bath pillow. Get a tall glass of ice water with lemon to keep yourself hydrated.

2. Then draw your bath...but not too hot (high temperatures are dangerous during pregnancy).

3. Add rose petals to uplift your mood or lemon slices to refresh and stimulate your senses. Use a few drops of essential oils—bergamot, chamomile, or lavender—to help you relax.

(Caution: The oils we recommend are safe to use, but certain essential oils are contraindicated during pregnancy. Please check with your healthcare provider before experimenting.)

4. Now, step in. Lie back, close your eyes, and release yourself from the stresses of the day. Practice the slow breathing and relaxation techniques you have been learning in your childbirth classes. Then look at your belly rising above the water. Enjoy its roundness. Watch the water ripple as your baby kicks....

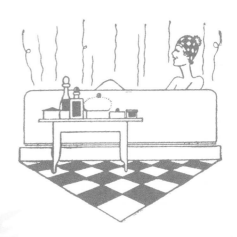

The Ultimate Facial

A soothing facial includes four key factors: steaming, cleaning, toning, and moisturizing. *Note*: Our cleanser doubles as an exfoliant.

STEAM: Soak a hand towel in a bowl of warm chamomile tea. Wrap the towel on your face and neck and leave it until cool. Repeat if desired. This process will open up pores for deeper cleansing. (Reserve some tea for the next step.)

CLEANSE & EXFOLIATE: Apply our Chamomile and Oats Cleanser/Exfoliant (see recipe below) in upward circular motions to stimulate skin and work out dirt and oil. Rinse thoroughly with warm water and pat face dry.

TONE: Soak a cotton ball with Rosewater Toner (see recipe on next page.) Gently pat the toner all over your face and neck. Don't rub. Leave to dry naturally.

MOISTURIZE: While your skin is still damp from the toner, apply a generous amount of 100 percent aloe vera gel to your face and neck. Let it soak in for 2–3 minutes before removing any excess gel with a soft tissue. For very dry spots, use small drops of pure Vitamin E.

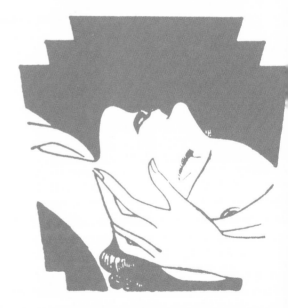

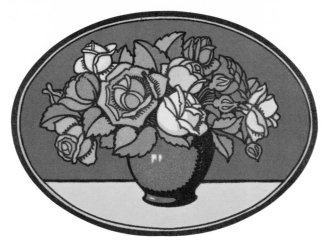

Recipes:

Chamomile and Oatmeal Cleanser/Exfoliant

2 tablespoons brewed chamomile tea (reserved from STEAM step)

1 tablespoon finely ground oats

1 tablespoon finely ground almonds

1 teaspoon honey

1 tablespoon 100% aloe vera gel

Combine all ingredients in a bowl and stir until well mixed.

Rosewater Toner

3 large handfuls fresh red rose petals

1 quart distilled water

1 sterile storage bottle

1. Place rose petals in a small saucepan.

2. Pour distilled water over petals and simmer on low heat until half the water is absorbed.

3. Allow the water to cool before discarding the petals. Pour the rosewater into the sterile storage bottle.

All these changes—some are wondrous, but some are a pain in the neck! Or is it your back? Actually it's more of a leg cramp....Well, it's no secret that as your baby grows and your body prepares for delivery, you'll experience some brand-new aches and pains. The good news is that with extra attention and care, you can work to prevent or assuage many of your pangs.

Oh, My Aching Back

Most pregnant women experience backaches, especially during the last trimester. As your pregnancy progresses, the increasing weight of your baby changes your center of gravity. To maintain balance, you may tend to arch your neck, pull back your shoulders, and push your belly forward.

Home Remedies: *Aches & Pains*

Unfortunately, these adjustments can greatly strain your back muscles. In addition, your body produces pregnancy hormones that start softening up ligaments, loosening up the spine and pelvis and preparing for the birth of the baby. Your destabilized pelvis can add to lower back strain.

So read through our tips, consider your changing body, and give some support to your poor aching back. And if your pain is continuous, severe, or runs down your leg toward your foot, be sure to consult your caregiver—a slipped disc can be serious business!

- Practice good posture by holding your spine straight when walking or standing. Try not to slouch and don't stand for too long. When standing, relieve stress by standing on a cushioned mat or with one foot up on a stool.

- When seated, sit with your back straight, your buttocks all the way to the back of the chair, and, if possible, your legs slightly elevated. Use chair arms to help you get up and avoid unsupportive, overly-cushioned, or backless chairs.

- Resist the urge to cross your legs while sitting. It can cause circulation troubles and exacerbate back problems by overly tilting your pelvis. Believe it or not, sitting can strain your back more than almost any other activity. Don't sit for too long—every 30 minutes, get up and stretch or take a short walk.

- Avoid bending forward, reaching high over your head, or making sudden, jerky movements.

- Learn to lift properly. Squat down, bending your knees and hips and keeping your back vertical. Grasp the item, close to your body, and slowly stand, lifting with your leg muscles, never bending at your waist. Avoid picking up heavy items, especially after your first trimester, and don't be shy about asking for help.

- Wear comfortable, low-heeled shoes that offer good support. Ask your caregiver or shoe salesperson about supportive inserts or shoes designed for extra comfort.

- Sleep on a firm, quality mattress with pillows supporting your legs and back. If your mattress is too soft, try placing a board under it. In the morning, slide your legs over the side of the bed and push yourself up into a sitting position.

- Relieve aching muscles with a warm bath in the morning and at night.

- Try to keep your weight within the recommended range to help ease the load on your back.

- Talk to your caregiver about supporting your back with a pregnancy girdle or a crisscross belly-support sling.

Ye-ouch — Charley Horse!

If you've ever had a cramp, or "charley horse," you know it's a sharply painful muscle spasm and it's certainly no fun. Cramps during pregnancy are often triggered by fatigue, changes in circulation, the additional weight you're carrying, or holding your body in a tense, awkward position. Leg and foot cramps are very common, especially at night during your last trimester, when you're trying to get some much-needed shuteye. And though the painful spasms usually last for only a moment, the affected muscle may continue to ache for some time after.

Thankfully, cramps often can be prevented or quickly soothed; if they continuously plague you, though, be sure to talk to your caregiver about solutions. Infrequently, a cramp may signify a blood clot, which is a serious medical condition.

Here are some suggestions to keep that mean charley horse at bay:

- If you elect to exercise during your pregnancy, always do a thorough warm-up and stretch for at least 15 minutes beforehand.

- Make sure to drink plenty of water and other fluids throughout the day.

- Try wearing support hose.

- Be sure to take breaks during the day, resting with your feet elevated.

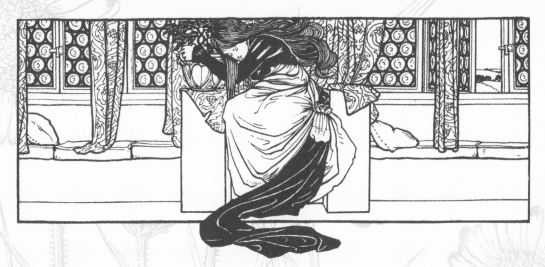

But if a charley horse gives you a good kick:

- Firmly massage the cramping muscle. Gently stretch your calf by flexing your foot, bringing your toes toward your face and pushing your heels down.

- For a more strenuous stretch, stand a half foot back from the wall or a sturdy chair. Put your hands on the wall or grip the back of the chair and slowly slide the cramping leg back, keeping your leg straight and your heel on the floor. Bend your other knee as you slide. Slide your leg back in and repeat as necessary.

- Flexing your feet and stretching your calves before bed may help prevent nighttime cramps.

- Use a warm compress to enhance your circulation and relieve the cramp.

- Some say that standing on a cold floor can help ease cramping.

Twins!

One lump or two? If it were this easy to predict the birth of twins, Old Wives wouldn't have much bothered. But as it were, they had many opinions. Rumor had it that twins always skipped generations. We now know that 2-egg twin tendencies are passed down from generation to generation through female lines and that approximately 1 in 43 pregnancies will be with twins.

Of course, twins are ultimately created when two separate eggs are fertilized, as in fraternal twins, or when a single egg divides as in identical twins. But according to the Wives, you can encourage twin production. If you and your husband made love twice while conceiving, twins are on the way. Do you enjoy the movies? Couples who took in a movie within three days of marriage are said to yield twins. And how about swimming? If you went swimming the day after your wedding, you're also assured of a "two-fer." Now look at your belly. Do you notice a red streak running down the middle? Another "twin sign"!

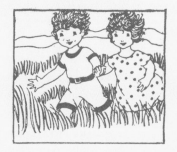

But this is not to say you shouldn't trust certain maternal instincts. Studies have shown that expectant mothers can intuitively identify the presence of multiples up to three months before the medical professionals can!

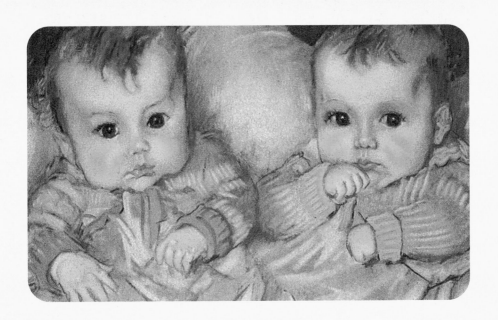

If you *are* having twins, you'll hear plenty more tales. Some say there's always a good twin and a bad twin or that the older twin will be a leader and the younger a follower. But don't bank on it–just when you think you've got your twins pigeonholed, they're likely to switch roles or join forces for more effective mischief-making. You also needn't worry about telling them apart. Even identical twins look subtly different, and all twins have their own distinctive personalities.

So when your great aunt breaks out the tea leaves and wonders, "One lump or two?" let's hope she's asking about sugar cubes. Unless she's picking up some of that mythical twins' ESP, your great aunt's got nothing on your caregiver!

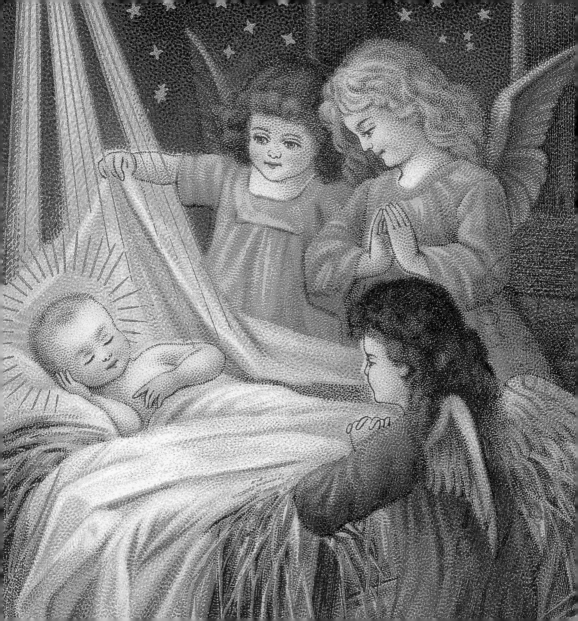

TRADITIONS: *Blessings*

Your new baby will be a blessing to you and your family. It's natural, in turn, to bless your baby at birth. In many cultures, blessings are part of a welcoming ceremony such as a bris or a baptism. Blessings also can simply be the first words that parents, family, and spiritual leaders say to newborns.

During the bris, when Jewish sons are circumcised, the father names his child and recites this blessing: "May the child [his name] grow up to Torah, to the wedding canopy and good deeds." Family and friends often express hopes that the baby was born under a good sign ("be-siman tov") or lucky star ("be-mazal tov"). Christians baptize their children to wash away "original sin" and bless them with a fresh beginning. Orthodox Christian babies are completely immersed in water three times. Roman Catholics and Anglicans anoint the baby's brow with a little water and mark a cross. In Senegal during a baby's naming ceremony, paper upon which prayers have been copied from the Koran is soaked in water. Then, before the infant is named, small pieces of the blessed paper are ripped off and placed on the baby's tongue.

The Orkney Islands offer a different take on ceremonies and blessings. After the baby is born, parents give out *blide-maet*, or "joy-food," at a feast held so friends and family can come and praise the baby and mother.

Any uttered admiration of the baby must be followed by "Guid save hid" (God save it) or "Sef bae hid" (Safe be it); otherwise, evil spirits might show unwanted attention, thinking the child too precious to live.

But a formal ceremony is not needed to bless a child. In many cultures, simple blessings are expressed by family and spiritual leaders when a baby is born. Mothers from Yemen might murmur to their infants, "My little meat, my little fat, my little honey, my grasshopper, my tiny moon, light of my eyes." Algiers midwives say, "I take the thorns from your path," three times as they pull imaginary thorns from the newborn's feet. The first words many Sikh parents utter to their babies are called the Mool Mantra:

> There is one God, Eternal truth is his name; He made everything
> and is in everything. He is not afraid of anything and is not
> fighting anything; He is not affected by time; He was not born,
> He made Himself; we know about Him from the teachings of the Guru.

A Muslim father greets his newborn by whispering the Call to Prayer, or *Adhan*, first in his child's right ear and then in the left. During birth, Navajos traditionally chant "The Blessing Way," a song meant to set the infant on a balanced, healthy, successful life path. After babies are born to Buddhist families, monks often attend the house, chanting and blessing the infant.

You will choose how you want to bless your baby. Whether it's part of a formal ceremony or just something quiet between you and your newborn, take the time to express your feelings, hopes, and prayers. And may your little blessing be forever blessed.

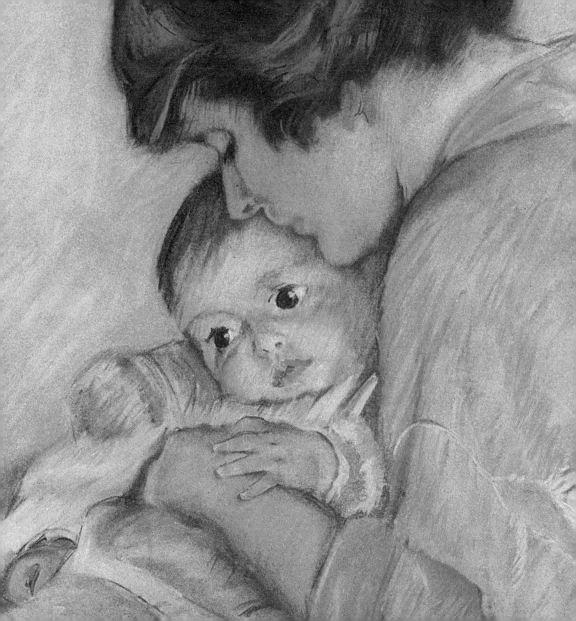

SATISFYING SANDWICHES

Varying your food choices at lunchtime can help take the monotony out of your meal and ensure that you and baby get lots of different nutrients. Try to eliminate favorite fallbacks such as processed meats, white breads, chips, cookies, and sodas as they are often high in sodium, sugar, and fat, and provide you with empty calories. Opt instead for fresh vegetables, whole-grain breads, and low-fat cheeses. Since sandwiches are a great way to pack a lot of nutrition into one easy-to-make meal, we came up with a few delicious suggestions.

BANANA NUTWICH

(Benefits: This easy-to-create sandwich satisfies both increased protein and potassium requirements for you and your baby, and can do wonders for curing a sweet tooth.)

Ingredients
¼ cup reduced-fat, low-sugar peanut butter

1 ripe banana, sliced

2 slices of whole-wheat bread, toasted

1. Spread half the peanut butter on each slice of toasted bread.

2. Top one side with banana, and place the other slice of toast on top. Cut sandwich in half, and serve.

Serves 1.

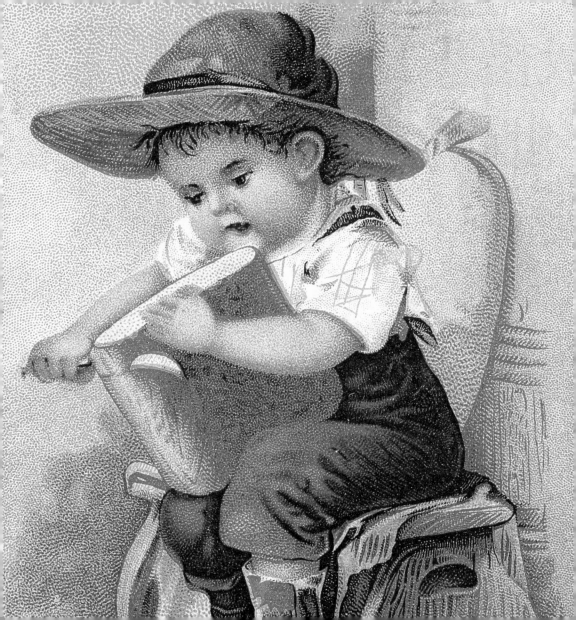

SATISFYING SANDWICHES

EGG SALAD PITA

(Benefits: This yummy protein booster is also good
served on rye crackers or as a side salad.)

Ingredients

4 eggs

1 celery stalk

2 tablespoons diced
dill pickle

2 tablespoons chopped
fresh dill

1 tablespoon reduced-fat
mayonnaise

1 teaspoon Dijon mustard

2 whole-wheat pita
pockets, cut in half

1. Place eggs in a pot with enough cold water to cover. Bring water to a boil, lower the heat, and simmer for about 10 minutes.

2. Dice the celery and combine it with the diced pickle and chopped dill.

3. Drain eggs and immediately submerge them in very cold water to cool before peeling. Chop two of the eggs and the other two egg whites, and add them to the celery mixture (discard extra yolks).

4. Stir in the mayonnaise and mustard, and mix well.

5. Chill mixture for 20 minutes or more.

6. Divide salad between pita pockets and serve.

Serves 2.

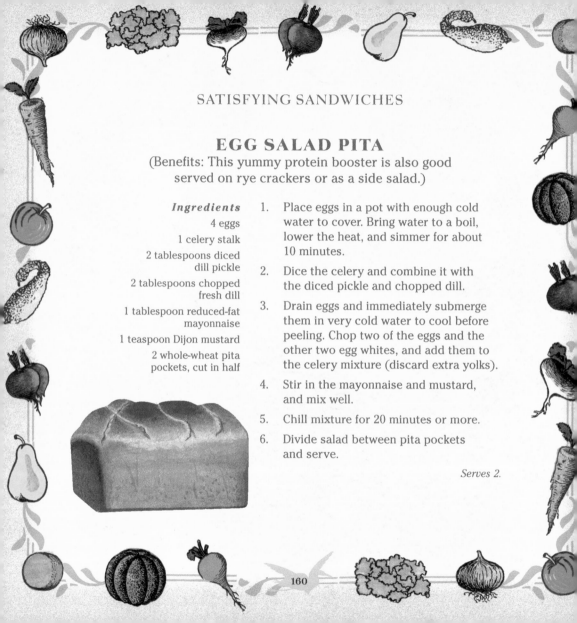

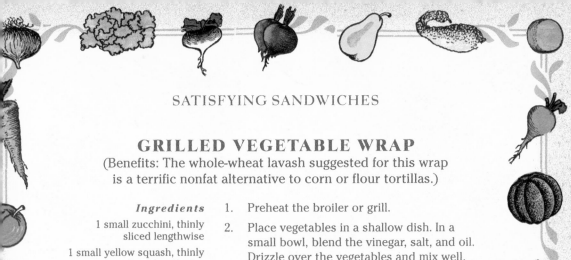

GRILLED VEGETABLE WRAP

(Benefits: The whole-wheat lavash suggested for this wrap
is a terrific nonfat alternative to corn or flour tortillas.)

Ingredients

1 small zucchini, thinly
sliced lengthwise

1 small yellow squash, thinly
sliced lengthwise

1 small red bell pepper,
cut into small strips

8 asparagus spears, tough
ends removed

$\frac{1}{2}$ teaspoon balsamic vinegar

Pinch kosher salt

1 teaspoon olive oil

$\frac{1}{4}$ cup pasteurized goat cheese

$\frac{1}{4}$ cup fat-free cream cheese

2 half sheets whole-wheat lavash

$\frac{1}{2}$ cup watercress leaves

1. Preheat the broiler or grill.

2. Place vegetables in a shallow dish. In a small bowl, blend the vinegar, salt, and oil. Drizzle over the vegetables and mix well. Set aside to marinate.

3. In another small bowl, combine the goat and cream cheeses.

4. Grill or broil vegetables until they can be pierced easily by a fork. Remove from heat and set aside.

5. Spread half the cheese mixture on each of the lavash halves. Layer the grilled vegetables and watercress on one end of the lavash. Roll the lavash tightly around the filling, and continue to fill the rest, tucking as you roll.

6. Cut each wrap in half on the diagonal, and serve.

Serves 2.

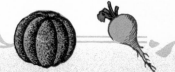

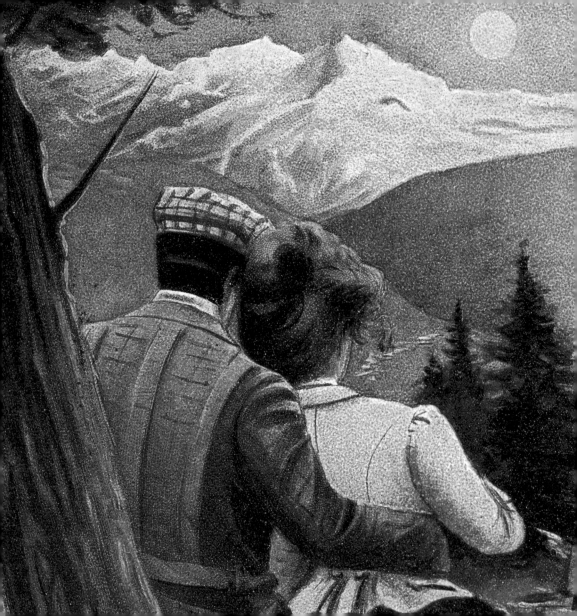

Spittin' Image

Rita Ciresi

I'M FROM CONNECTICUT; my husband is from California. We've never visited Oklahoma, but it's our favorite musical—especially the number in which Ado Annie, the Girl Who Can't Say No, finally decides to put a halt to her flirting and accepts Cowboy Will's marriage proposal with the coy line, "Supposing that we should have a third one?" and Will warns, "He better look a lot like me."

After Ado Annie swears, "Da spittin' image!" I always try to imagine actually *wanting* a child who would resemble me. Neither my husband nor I is considered radically ugly, but we aren't conventionally beautiful either, and our looks clearly don't "match."

I've got nothing against my genes or my husband's, but I'm sure once they get mixed up, the result will be goofy stuff.

We were living in central Pennsylvania (appropriately surrounded by fecund acres of feed corn and lowing Holstein cows) when I get pregnant. When we hesitantly approach the contraception counter at Fay's Drug to buy a pregnancy test, we also buy, on impulse, five lottery tickets. When

Spittin' Image

the stick turns pink (and our numbers fail to hit), we immediately start speculating on yet another wild shot at the jackpot: the chances of our baby winning any kind of beauty contest.

"Purty slim," I tell my husband.

He shrugs. "All babies are supposed to look like Winston Churchill."

"All WASP babies, maybe," I say glumly, sure ours will look like either Mussolini or Golda Meir.

"Do you suppose it'll have red hair?" my husband asks, knowing that once upon a time, we both had so much brass on our heads we were the butt of many a milkman joke. "What if it really does look like me?"

"Or *moi*," says I. "Even worse: What if it looks like both of us?"

We buy more lottery tickets and start saving for a nose job. For the baby, that is.

By now you will have guessed: In both our families, a good schnozz is not hard to find. To locate a magazine-pretty face—American-style—we might have to beat the bushes all the way back to Adam and Eve.

I descend—and I'm afraid, *look* like it—from a long line of ragpickers, cigar rollers, piano polishers, and spindle operators in the Smoothee Foundation Factory. I had foolish hopes that college would function as a sort of plastic surgery. For me to keep such a remarkable resemblance—

Spittin' Image

after earning a B.A. and two graduate degrees—to a great-uncle who for fifty years stood on an assembly line attaching straps to bathing caps seems a dire fate indeed.

After I get pregnant, I stare for hours at the dozens of photographs of my solemn ancestors and the very few pictures that remain of the forebears on my husband's side.

Individual photos in the family album show smiling boys in knickers and sailor hats ready to visit the 1939 World's Fair; a girl in a drop-waist dress posed on a pony at Coney Island. Hard to believe—or all to easy to imagine—the fate of this happy little girl had her grandfather not emigrated at the turn of the century. Her pretty blond curls, ashes. The delicate locket around her neck melted for the gold.

The war between our genes, fought in a split-second blaze of glory as the sperm collided with the ovum, inevitably was a nasty thing, and I have nine long months to speculate on its various foul outcomes: male pattern baldness. Long-lobed ears that produce too much wax. Wrinkles that cross thick necks like multistrand chokers. Knock knees that creak when you walk up the stairs. Toes that curl more than your hair. Short waists. Withered elbows. Deep bruises beneath the eyes. Double chins. Triple chins. Low hairlines. Ridged fingernails. Hairy nostrils. Hairy legs and hairy chests. Hairy everything!

Spittin' Image

"At least we're both skinny," I tell my husband, conveniently forgetting for a moment that there were so many obese folks in our family that my sister and I once concocted an entertainment called "The Fat Relatives Game." This amusement ran along the lines of "Twenty Questions," and was played only in bed, out of earshot of our parents.

"Actually—I ought to tell you—you really should know—that a lot of people in my family were like—kind of plump," I admit to my husband as we sit at Hoss's Steak House, where my plate reflects the awful bottomless pit of hunger and wild, disgusting cravings I will suffer from during my entire pregnancy and, alas, far beyond: an eight-ounce bloody steak, a baked potato with a big ball of butter, half a loaf of garlic bread and—still left over from my second trip to the all-you-can-eat salad bar—macaroni and peas and hard-boiled eggs, black olives and bacon bits, and enough sunflower seeds to feed a flock of parakeets for a year.

"Like who?" my husband says. "Who's plump?"

"They're all dead now."

I eat some more. A lot more. Then I ask, "What do people die of in your family?"

"Cancer. And yours?"

"Strokes and heart attacks."

He reaches across the table and scoops the butter out of my potato. I confiscate the steak sauce—the fine print on the label informs me it's loaded with preservatives.

Spittin' Image

Oh, what a meal! The baby burps and hiccups all night.

My pregnancy books—which are supposed to calm my fears, but do
nothing more than fan the flames of my neurosis—demonstrate in monthly
charts the progression of fetal growth, from a black speck of caviar to a
squirmy tadpole, to a Jacques Cousteau frogman, to a translucent monkey
sucking its thumb and strumming its penis like there's no tomorrow. Right
around the Dr. Seuss's Star-Bellied Sneetch stage, I get an ultrasound,
which makes me even more wigged out, not about the baby, but about my
incredibly weak bladder, which feels poised to explode after drinking
thirty-two ounces of liquid an hour before.

"Here we are," the technician announces, positioning the monitor on
my stomach and turning the screen toward me to display a wide, almost
evil face, spooky white against the black background, a couple of paws
clenched against her body, and two trundle-bed legs with—thank God!—
none of that tiresome peeny-weeny stuff in between.

"It's a girl!" the technician announces.

Like your average mall rat, she's just hanging out—not doing anything
to indicate she's Harvard material. Then with one tiny fist she reaches up
and—waves at us!

She's a genius. She's the gal I love. She's the most beautiful girl I've
ever seen.

Spittin' Image

Writers are supposed to have fertile, perverted imaginations. Why, then, after seeing You (for after having been mugged on the sonogram, the Baby has become flesh and blood, a real entity capable of being addressed in the second person)—why can I only imagine You in a lifetime of the most middle-of-the-road situations, smiling your Kodak grin as I take endless shots of your life like a photographer searching for the perfect moment? All right, it's barf city—the most sentimental hogwash on the planet—but I picture you prancing in your first pink tutu, playing *Für Elise* on the piano, marching down the aisle at your high school graduation, your mortarboard sitting cockily on your head to indicate it's no sweat, baby, to be valedictorian. You are brilliant because you are homely. And because you're such a smarty-pants, you save me scads of money. You have a full scholarship to become the first female Whiffenpoof at Yale. You will be the best god-damn—well, *whatever*, as long as it's financially lucrative—on the East Coast, and support me in my old age as I try to write feeble essays such as this for a hundred dollars a pop (if I'm lucky). You have the same exact bra size as me. You say, "Mom, Tolstoy never made the best-seller list either." You say you hear the voice of God in every syllable of my penned words, and then you screech at me, "I'll never forget—never forgive you for—that time Grandma pointed at me and asked 'Is this child going to be Catholic or Jewish or—' and you answered, 'Just plain old fucked-up, I guess.'"

Spittin' Image

In the ninth month, the evil truth surfaces: My father-in-law has six toes.

"Six altogether?" I ask, horrified, and my husband says, "No, on one foot. I'm sure I've told you this before. He's got a toe extra."

The logistics of this are beyond me. How does my father-in-law find shoes to fit? Does he have to admit to this deformity to those smarmy salesmen in the white shirts at Standard Shoes who ask "What size, sir?" Does he feel empowered by his extra toe? What if he had an extra finger? No wonder he doesn't like to go to the beach.

This news inspires me with such wonder, terror, and dread that I have to go to bed early just to forget about it. I wake at midnight, thinking, "Jeez, my stomach hurts." Then, glancing around the dark room and barely making out the faint outline of the empty crib in the corner, I remember I'm full term. Four days overdue. And I think, "Jeez, sure would be nice to get some sleep." But you, Baby Cakes, are determined not to give me a wink of it, as if to prepare me for all the sleepless nights to come.

We drive to the hospital. Three hours into labor I get a shot of Demerol to take away the pain, which causes me to vomit, and makes me drift off into half-sleep.

"Are you ready to push?" the nurse asks, and, taken by my pain back to some preverbal state, I grunt and snort, which she—experienced at this sort of thing—knows how to translate into a firm *yes-sirree, ma'am!* The

Spittin' Image

bottom half of the bed is unlocked and rolled away. The nurse points to the mirror in the corner of the room, a convex affair that reminds me of the kind our local pharmacist used to glance into to make sure we deprived neighborhood kids weren't stealing Smartees and petal-pink Maybelline nail polish from his drugstore.

"Watch your baby being born!" the nurse urges me.

"Fuck you!" I holler. Then: "Take it out!"

"Push it out!" she commands me, and I squirt seven pounds of blood, sweat, and tears into the doctor's hands.

"You have a beautiful baby girl," the doctor announces and plops the shivering red bundle, still attached by a pulsing, bulbous umbilical cord, on my belly. The rude, squinched face of a succubus stares up at me, and then Baby Cakes lets out a tongue-vibrating cry. *Well*, I think, *I'd scream if I looked like that, too.* Consumed with love and repulsion—and my first maternal impulse, the urge to say "Go get yourself washed and clean, and don't let me see such a filthy little face again, young lady!"—I repeat, "Take it away!" and after a quick clip of the cord, the nurse makes a move on my progeny.

"How many toes does she have?" I ask my husband, after they take Baby over to the sink to clean her up and bundle her into her heated crib. My husband doesn't look at me. He doesn't even answer me. He's got a new love, now. Might as well get used to it.

Spittin' Image

"Ten," the nurse says. "I always count them."

Later she gives me a sponge bath and takes me back to my room in a wheelchair. "So what do you think of your baby?" she asks, and I have to admit I can hardly even remember those brief moments they let me hold her in my arms, except the uncanny replication of my mother-in-law's nose, my father-in-law's ears, and my husband's cute cowlick on her pookie little head.

"She looks exactly like my husband's side of the family," I say.

"They always look like their dads at first," the nurse says. "It's Darwinian. I guess it kept cavemen from accusing their women of being unfaithful and dashing their children to bits against the walls of the cave."

I pause. "You'd think men would have gotten over that by now."

"You would have thought so, yes," she says.

And now it's just Beautiful You and Fat Relative Me, kid. On the first clear, sunny day after we're home from the hospital, I bundle you in your bonnet and bunting and take you out for a stroll in your spanking new blue carriage, feeling oddly like an eight-year-old girl pushing her new Pee-and-Pop Dolly down the street. As I command the stroller toward the country club, wincing (will my stitches never heal?), I look into your wet brown eyes, which are about as Sicilian-looking as a chocolate *biscotto* dunked in *cafe latte*—and

Spittin' Image

about as far from those blue eyes of my husband's family as you can get. Your smooth cheeks are so intensely pale, I vow to buy stock in Banana Boat, knowing the company is going to make a mint off the amount of sunscreen both of us will have to apply to ward off the burns and moles that could ruin our too-white skin.

I stop the stroller on the ninth green of the golf course, and lift you up so you can see, for the first time, this mindless addictive sport that I pray you will not engage in when you retire. "Mine," I murmur, as I hold your cheek against my face. "You're all mine."

Two older women stand on the green. One turns her gaze away from the tee and looks over at us. "What a pretty little girl!" she calls out to me, looking from the baby's cap of blond curls to my dark mop. "Is she adopted?"

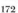

172

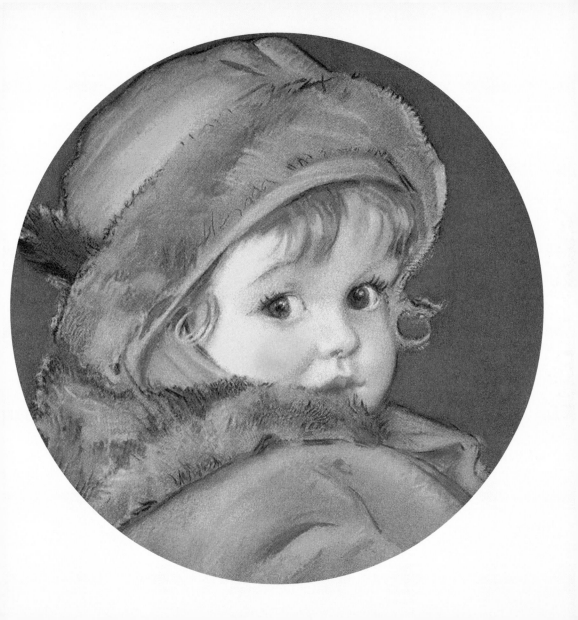

Your Baby's Character

Nine months can be a long time. During this period, you'll have plenty of hours to daydream and wonder what kind of person your baby will be. Will your child be strong? Generous? Prosperous? Patient...? In case *you* are not so patient, we've polled the Old Wives and compiled some sayings that might help you influence and predict your baby's nature. Keep in mind, of course, that nature alone will have the ultimate say!

Numerous cultures believe your behavior during pregnancy can affect your child's, sex, character and physical well-being, especially when it comes to what you eat or *don't* eat. The Chinese have always believed you can influence the sex of your baby by consuming certain kinds of foods for seven days before conceiving. For a boy, dine on carrots, lettuce, mushrooms, and tofu. For a girl, eat fish, meat, and pickles. Some Native American mothers-to-be avoid berries for fear of birthmarks, steelhead salmon for fear of babies with weak ankles, and seagulls or cranes for fear of "crybabies."

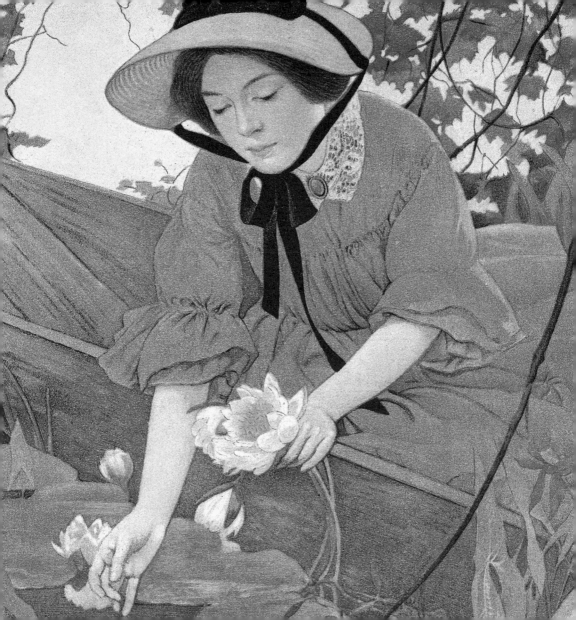

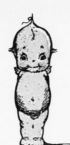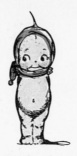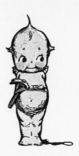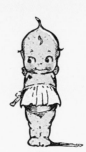

In Uganda, expectant mothers are told not to drink water while standing so their babies won't be born with squinted eyes.

If you're a believer, you'll also want to be aware of these unusual superstitions: The Aztecs believed that a pregnant woman who saw an eclipse would have a baby with a harelip; in China, a mother-to-be who rubs her belly too much might produce a spoiled, over-demanding child; and general folk wisdom asserts that happily married couples will have good-looking children, while the babies of couples who argue are fated to be less than attractive.

Some cultures say the timing of your baby's birth offers insights. In China, the hour, day, month, and year of childbirth decide which of Eight Characters the baby is born under. The Character then helps determine the baby's future success, wealth, and good fortune.

Another superstition asserts that a baby born on Sunday cannot be harmed by evil spirits. In Malta, many believe a boy born on Saint Mary's Day in August will become a great horse racer. And some say that a baby born at night will stay awake at night.

So once your baby arrives, what can you predict about personality? It is said a baby that emerges feet first will have healing abilities. A baby born

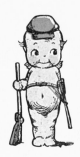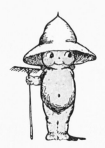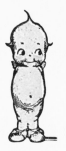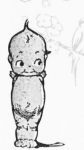

from a red water sac is believed to have great powers and double sight. Large ears foretell your baby will be generous. If your baby is born with open hands and out-stretched fingers, some see prosperity. A large mouth predicts a good singer (though beware—a baby born with teeth could grow up to be a vampire!) The Chinese say wide, thick ears or a concave navel are signs of future happiness and success. And when in doubt, parents in both China and Malta place symbolic objects like an ink well, needlework, a book, rosary beads, or an official seal in a basket and offer it to the baby. The first object the baby grabs signifies the child's destiny.

Still anxious? Well, perhaps you can influence characteristics even after your baby is born. In the Pacific's Caroline Islands, parents place the baby's umbilical cord in a conch shell they then use to influence the baby's future. For example, if parents think their child will one day need to be a good climber, they hang the conch on a tree. Germans say that a newborn laid first on her left side will grow up to be clumsy. Native American mothers were known to dunk male sons in water to assure they'd become strong, brave men and hardy hunters. And in China, rubbing a cooked chicken's tongue on your baby's lips is said to make your child a good talker.

And you have dreams about your kids. You have dreams that maybe one day your kid will be up there saying, "I'd like to thank the Nobel Academy..." Then you have this other dream where your kid is going, "Ya want fries with this?"

–Robin Williams

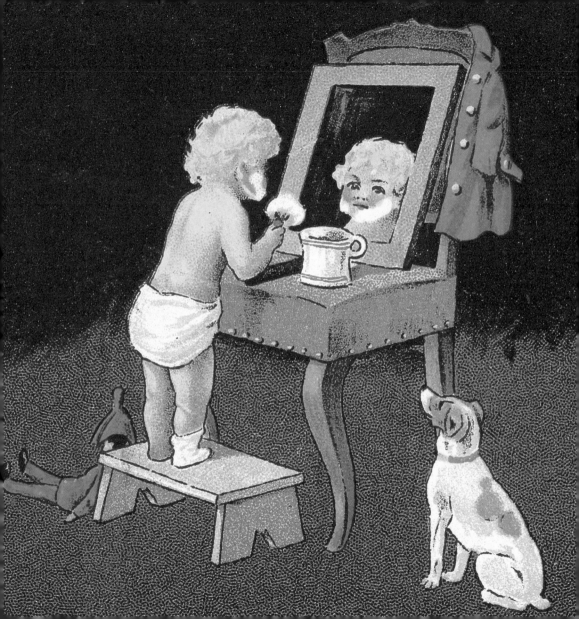

BIRTHDAY FACTS

Month	Zodiac Sign	Birth Stone
JANUARY	Capricorn (Dec. 22 – Jan. 19)	Garnet
FEBRUARY	Aquarius (Jan. 20 – Feb. 18)	Amethyst
MARCH	Pisces (Feb. 19 – Mar. 20)	Aquamarine
APRIL	Aries (Mar. 21 – Apr. 19)	Diamond
MAY	Taurus (Apr. 20 – May 20)	Emerald
JUNE	Gemini (May 21 – June 21)	Pearl
JULY	Cancer (June 22 – July 22)	Ruby
AUGUST	Leo (July 23 – Aug. 22)	Peridot
SEPTEMBER	Virgo (Aug. 23 – Sept. 22)	Sapphire
OCTOBER	Libra (Sept. 23 – Oct. 22)	Opal
NOVEMBER	Scorpio (Oct. 23 – Nov. 21)	Topaz
DECEMBER	Sagittarius (Nov. 22 – Dec. 21)	Turquoise

STONE MEANING	BIRTH FLOWER	FLOWER MEANING
Constancy	White carnation	Pure love
Sincerity	Violet	Modesty, virtue, faithfulness
Courage	Daffodil, Jonquil	Respect, chivalry
Innocence	Sweet Pea	Blissful pleasures
Success	Lily of the valley	Sweetness
Longevity	Rose	Beauty of youth
Contentment	Larkspur	Open heart
Happiness	Gladiolas	Strength of character
Clear thinking	Aster	Enthusiasm
Hope	Marigold	Sacred affection
Fidelity	Chrysanthemum	Long life
Prosperity	Paperwhite	Female ambition

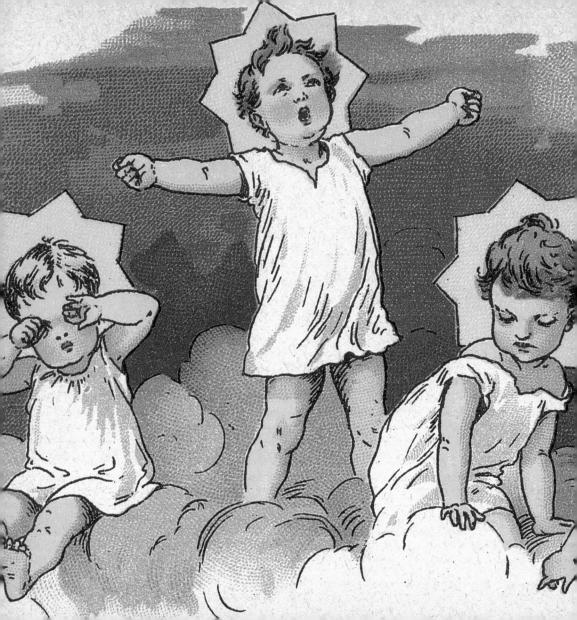

Monday's Child

Monday's child is fair of face,
Tuesday's child is full of grace,
Wednesday's child is full of woe,
Thursday's child has far to go,
Friday's child is loving and giving,
Saturday's child works hard for its living,
But the child that is born on the Sabbath day
Is bonny, and blithe, and good, and gay.

Creating Community

Let's face it—pregnancy and parenting (especially first-time parenting) can be isolating. Some of your "friends" may have no interest in changing their lifestyle to hang out with a momma-to-be, even a chic one. Other pals, whom you've relied on for advice about dating, work, and your hair, may find it increasingly difficult to relate to your new concerns—heartburn, the nursery décor, and episiotomies.

Finding or creating your own support network during pregnancy is a vital factor in maintaining sanity. Having a group of friendly ears to share common concerns, emotions, and milestones with can be a great source of comfort and joy. So get out there and mingle! Life's too short to stay indoors with the shades down. But where to start? Here are a few suggestions:

◆ Make an effort to meet and exchange numbers with other participants in your childbirth classes.

◆ Contact your local La Leche League for information about support groups for nursing mothers.

◆ Join a prenatal fitness class at your local YWCA or health club.

◆ Head out to the local park, playground, or coffee shop and connect with the people in your neighborhood.

◆ Seek out support group information on bulletin boards at nearby churches, community centers, or in the community paper.

◆ Advertise your own group for pregnant women and new mothers. Meet once a week for coffee, a potluck, or a walk in the park.

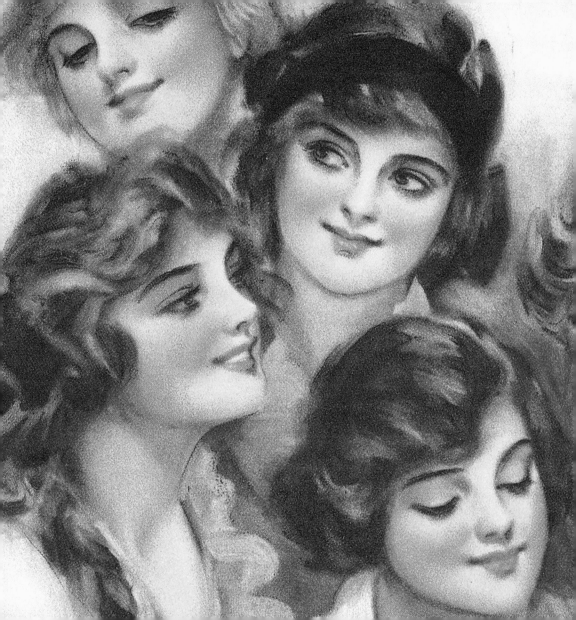

Kegel Exercises

What are they? What is the point? How do I do them? Kegel exercises are a muscle-group isolation technique that serves to tighten the pelvic floor muscles that support the urethra, bladder, uterus, and rectum. Strengthening the pelvic floor muscles will help you:

- maintain better bladder control during and after pregnancy

- improve sex for you and your partner during pregnancy and after delivery

- condition your body for an easier child-birth (fewer tears in the perineum)

The most important step in learning how to perform a Kegel is to identify the target muscles. Here is one simple way to do this. Contract your pelvic muscles as you would to stop the flow of urine. Repeat this a few times until you get the feel of isolating the correct muscle group. To practice a Kegel, contract the muscles for a count of 10–20 seconds, and then release for another few seconds. Repeat ten to twenty times. It is recommended that you perform the exercise two to three times a day. You can practice Kegels anywhere, anytime—no one will know but you!

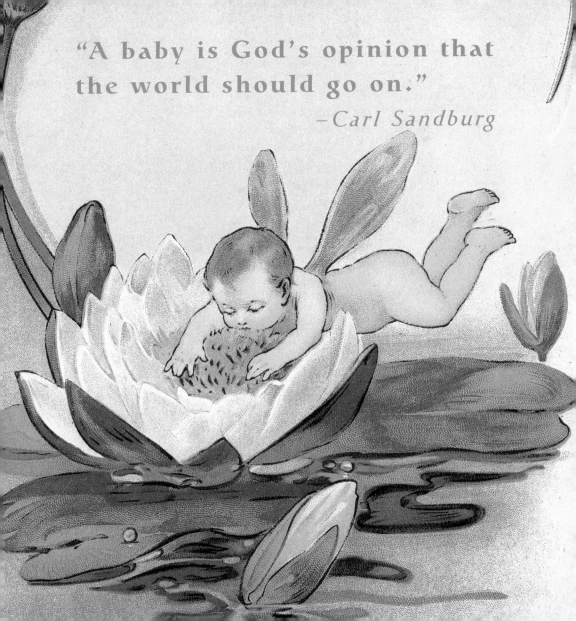

"A baby is God's opinion that the world should go on."

–Carl Sandburg

TRADITIONS: *Gift Giving*

In countries around the world it is customary to contribute to the health and happiness of the expectant family through the long-cherished tradition of gift giving. While presents and their purposes come in all shapes and sizes, they are always offered in love, respect, celebration, and good will.

Western families often throw parties for pregnant mothers—"showering" them with gifts for the coming baby, hence the name "baby shower." Other cultures have their own versions of this time-honored event. In numerous Indian states, a woman in her seventh month of pregnancy is feted by female relatives, who give her gifts; in Tamil Nadu, the woman's mother gives her a pair each of silver and gold bangles; and in Gujarat, the woman's mother-in-law puts coconut, money, and rice in the woman's lap, and they pass the presents back and forth seven times. Similarly, a Muslim custom dictates that, some time during the expectant mom's seventh or ninth month, she dresses in a new outfit and her friends and relatives fill her lap with fruits and vegetables. In China, a month before birth, the expectant woman's mother sends her daughter *tsue shen*, or "hastening the delivery" package, which contains white swaddling cloth. But many, including traditional Chinese and Jewish families, consider baby showers unlucky.

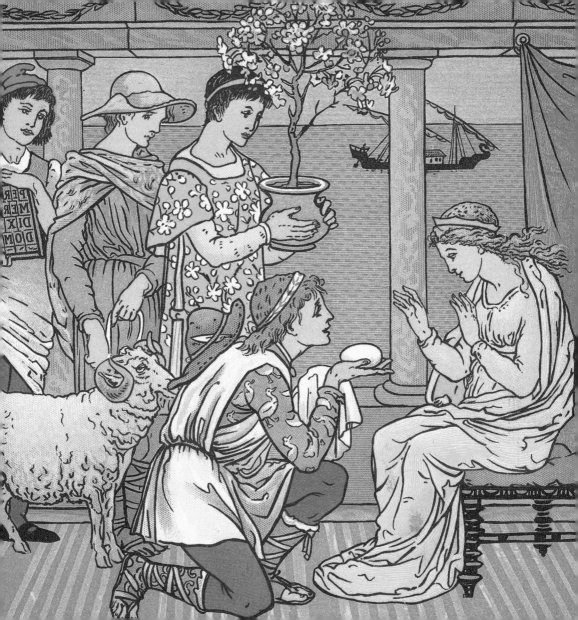

These aversions, formed in times when infant mortality rates were high, often involve fear of attracting evil spirits, jinxing happiness, or simply being overly presumptuous that humans can control fate.

After the baby is born, the gift giving begins in earnest. In Sikh families, the new mother's parents celebrate the first-born, especially if the child is a boy, by bringing over a package called *shushak*. The package contains a silver spoon, plate, bowl, and glass; clothes for the baby, the new father's family, and their servants; and—if they can afford it—a gold decoration and money for the new mother, mother-in-law, and baby. In China, on the third day after a birth, guests attend the infant's ceremonial first bath. Visitors put a colored egg or fruit into the bathwater, pour a spoonful of cold water into the wash-basin, and give the newborn a small silver present. On the baby's one-month birthday, he or she is feted with food and gifts. Close family and neighbors give baby clothes (often tiger-themed, since tigers are thought to protect children), red envelopes filled with money, and chicken essence for the new mom. In return, the guests get small red and yellow cakes and dyed-red hard-boiled eggs for good luck. Japanese parents bring their newborns to temples, where friends and family give them protective toy dogs and other presents.

Some gifts are given for special purposes or future ceremonies. In Japan, infant girls often receive papier-mâché totems called *inubariko*, which they keep by their bedside as they mature. When the young women marry, they take the totems with them as symbols of fertility and trouble-free childbirth. Ancient Romans gave nine-day-old infants boxes with charms (*bullas*) to

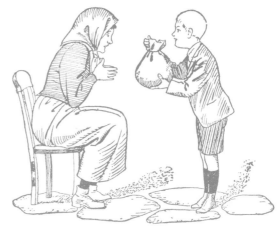

protect them from evil spirits. A custom that survives amongst the Baruya in New Guinea is the act of giving a newborn a bar of salt, which the family stores on the hearth and uses during the baby's naming ceremony.

If you're still wondering what to ask for or give in celebration of a birth, consider another age-old tradition. One of the five basic tenets of Muslim belief is *zakat*, or giving to those in need. In preparation for the Muslim naming ceremony, the infant's hair is shaved off and weighed. As a thank-you to God, the parents then give away the same weight, and usually more, in silver. What better way to celebrate a new baby, a most precious gift, than by giving to others?

Openings

Gayle Brandeis

WHEN I WAS PREGNANT the first time, my sister gave me a pendant. It was a circle, with a woman figure squatting inside. Her hands were raised over her head, and her birth canal was open—out, to the world; in, to her full, round womb.

I wore the pendant after my son was born, but I felt like I was cheating. My birth canal had not opened. Arin was born by emergency C-section after a scary transfer from the birth center to the hospital. Although I fully dilated, and pushed for over an hour, there was serious fetal distress, and the moment of birth was taken from me. I was unconscious, shut down, when Arin was delivered, and my body was stapled closed.

Three years later, pregnant again, I put the pendant back on. I was determined to have a vaginal birth after cesarean. I knew I could do it, but some scared, scarred, part of me had doubts that my body could open into birth.

Then, my friend Valarie showed up at my door. The sky was beginning to get dark, but the moon was full and radiant.

"We have to go somewhere," she said mysteriously.

I woke up my napping husband so he could watch Arin, and I let Valarie usher me into her car.

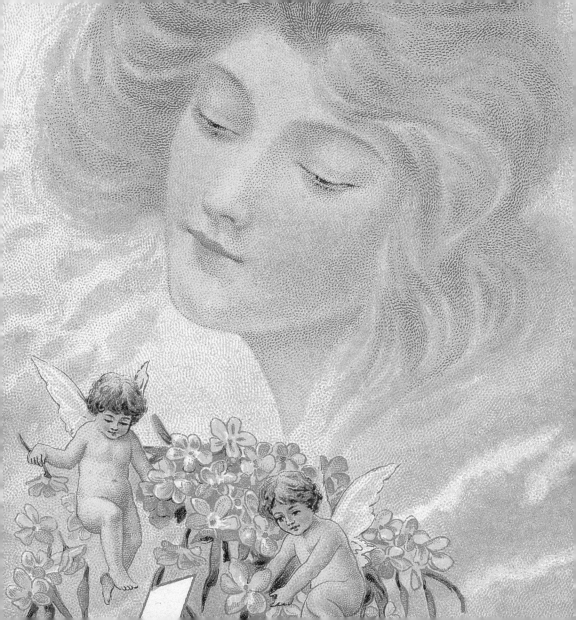

Openings

"Where are you taking me?" I asked. The street lamps lit up as we passed them.

She just smiled.

I sank back in the passenger seat, my eight-month big belly pointing toward the moon. This is like labor, I thought. You never know where it will take you. I decided to trust the journey, and enjoy the ride.

Valarie stopped the car, and we got out. As we walked across some grass, Valarie began to sing:

"I am opening, I am o-pen-ing…"

"This is a ceremony for you," she whispered between phrases. "A blessing way."

By a grove of trees in the distance, I saw a circle of flickering light. Flickering voices joined Valarie in song. I felt like I was entering sacred space. I walked toward the circle on dream legs.

Four women—Kate, Elisa, Debbie, Amy—sat holding candles. I was drawn into the circle. A blanket was wrapped around me. Someone removed my barrette and brushed my hair. My shoes were taken off, my feet bathed in a bowl of warm water and flower petals, then dusted with cornmeal. A wreath of leaves and berries was placed on my head.

A bowl of smoking sage was passed around the circle. Each woman brought the bowl to her eyes, for clear vision; to her mouth,

Openings

that her words may be true; her heart, for good sharing; her hands, to bless all the hands do; and her feet, that she may walk in a sacred way.

Valarie began to chant—Ya No Ho Wey Ya Ho Wey Ney—Gayle will birth like a bear, she said. Gayle will birth with the strength of a bear.

Together we breathed deep, let deep open sounds come from our throats. Together we drew power from the earth and each other.

Then, one by one, the women came up to me, holding candles. They each gave me a beautiful, heart-made gift, then joined their single candles' flames to the large candle in the center. They took their candles home with them so that when I went into labor, they could light them, to be with me in spirit, to help me blaze through the birth.

My heart opened that night, deep and wide. The Blessing Way, so unexpected, so magical, took me to a place of awe and gratitude. A place flew open so wide within myself, there were no words to express it. We didn't need words.

The opening woman is not honored in our culture. Baby showers are held, gifts are given, but the woman who opens her body is not acknowledged in any meaningful way. The Blessing Way, a Native

Openings

American tradition, truly honors the woman who opens her body to let life pass through. Traditional baby showers can also be transformed to empower the woman near her birthing time. At my baby shower, each woman brought a bead. Many of the beads had stories behind them: my mother-in-law gave me a bead her mother used to wear, my friend Kate gave me a shell she found on a beach in Baja when her son first weaned. We strung the beads together and created a necklace full of women, full of mother-energy.

One full-moon later, I put the necklace on again. My friends from the Blessing Way lit their candles. The labor was long and hard. I pushed for two hours without making much progress. The baby was stuck at my tailbone, the bone hooked in like a question mark, not letting her pass through. I got to a point where I wasn't sure I could push anymore. I thought I would have to be cut open again, unconscious, stapled shut.

And then, my body opened to the bear. Gayle will birth like a bear. Gayle will birth with the strength of a bear. Suddenly, my tired body was charged with bear muscle. I became the animal. A strength I did not know I had, blossomed from the center of my body.

"The channel's been opened," my midwife said.

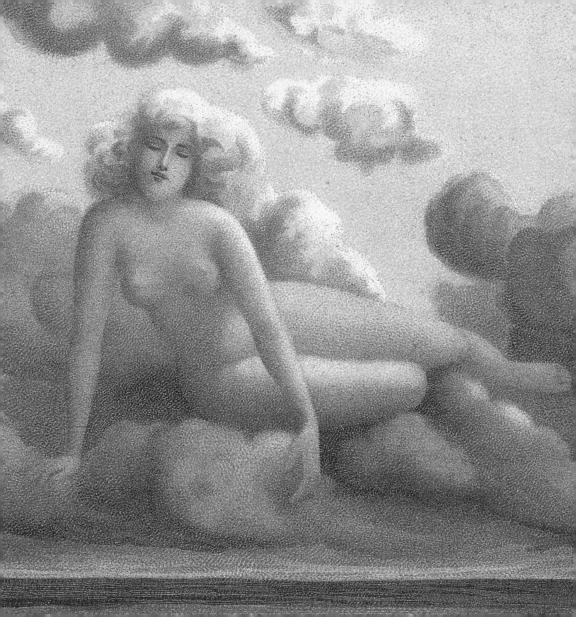

The Moment the Two Worlds Meet

Sharon Olds

That's the moment I always think of—when the
slick, whole body comes out of me,
when they pull it out, not pull it but steady it
as it pushes forth, not catch it,
    but steady it
as it pushes forth, not catch it but keep their
hands under it as it pulses out,
they are the first to touch it,
and it shines, it glistens with the thick liquid on it.
That's the moment, while it's sliding, the limbs
compressed close to the body, the arms
bent like a crab's rosy legs, the
thighs closely packed plums in heavy syrup, the
legs folded like the white wings of a chicken—
that is the center of life, that moment when the
juiced bluish sphere of the baby is
sliding between the two worlds,
wet, like sex, it *is* sex,
it is my life opening back and back
as you'd strip the reed from the bud, not strip it but
watch it thrust so it peels itself and the
flower is there, severely folded, and
then it begins to open and dry
but by then the moment is over,
they wipe off the grease and wrap the child in a blanket and
hand it to you entirely in this world.

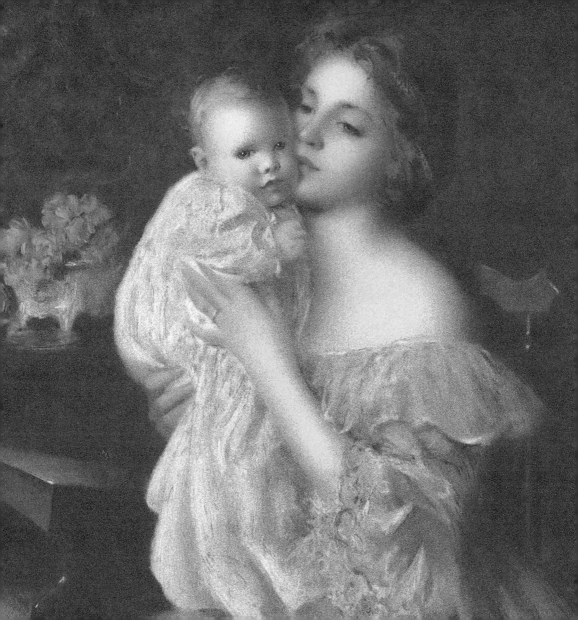

SUPER SALADS

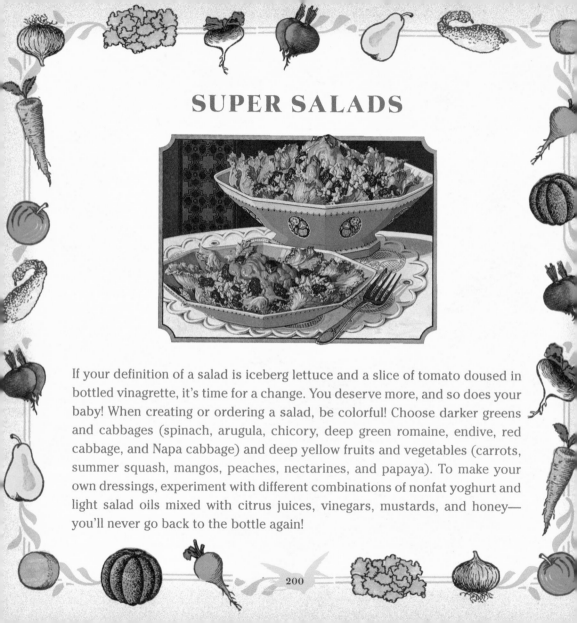

If your definition of a salad is iceberg lettuce and a slice of tomato doused in bottled vinagrette, it's time for a change. You deserve more, and so does your baby! When creating or ordering a salad, be colorful! Choose darker greens and cabbages (spinach, arugula, chicory, deep green romaine, endive, red cabbage, and Napa cabbage) and deep yellow fruits and vegetables (carrots, summer squash, mangos, peaches, nectarines, and papaya). To make your own dressings, experiment with different combinations of nonfat yoghurt and light salad oils mixed with citrus juices, vinegars, mustards, and honey— you'll never go back to the bottle again!

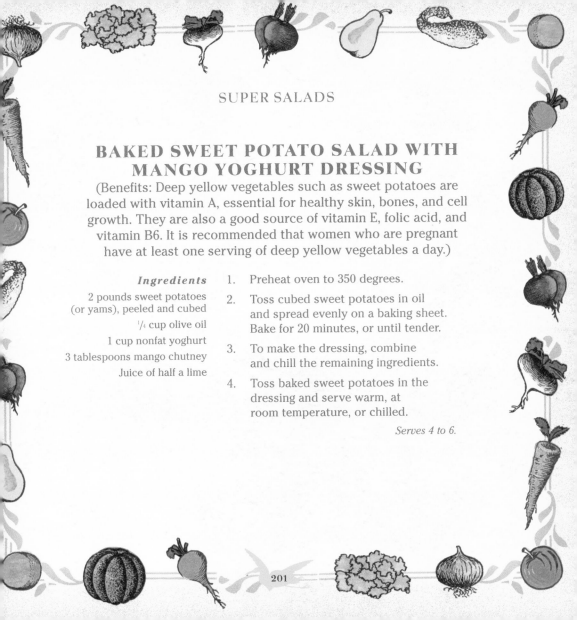

BAKED SWEET POTATO SALAD WITH MANGO YOGHURT DRESSING

(Benefits: Deep yellow vegetables such as sweet potatoes are loaded with vitamin A, essential for healthy skin, bones, and cell growth. They are also a good source of vitamin E, folic acid, and vitamin B6. It is recommended that women who are pregnant have at least one serving of deep yellow vegetables a day.)

Ingredients

2 pounds sweet potatoes
(or yams), peeled and cubed

¼ cup olive oil

1 cup nonfat yoghurt

3 tablespoons mango chutney

Juice of half a lime

1. Preheat oven to 350 degrees.

2. Toss cubed sweet potatoes in oil and spread evenly on a baking sheet. Bake for 20 minutes, or until tender.

3. To make the dressing, combine and chill the remaining ingredients.

4. Toss baked sweet potatoes in the dressing and serve warm, at room temperature, or chilled.

Serves 4 to 6.

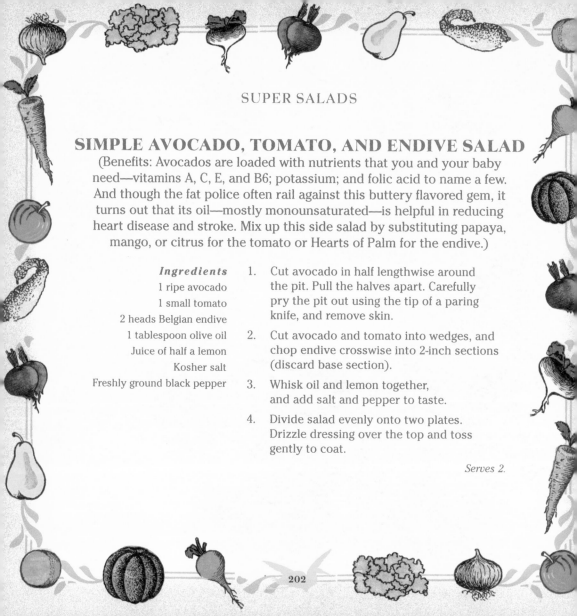

SIMPLE AVOCADO, TOMATO, AND ENDIVE SALAD

(Benefits: Avocados are loaded with nutrients that you and your baby need—vitamins A, C, E, and B6; potassium; and folic acid to name a few. And though the fat police often rail against this buttery flavored gem, it turns out that its oil—mostly monounsaturated—is helpful in reducing heart disease and stroke. Mix up this side salad by substituting papaya, mango, or citrus for the tomato or Hearts of Palm for the endive.)

Ingredients
1 ripe avocado
1 small tomato
2 heads Belgian endive
1 tablespoon olive oil
Juice of half a lemon
Kosher salt
Freshly ground black pepper

1. Cut avocado in half lengthwise around the pit. Pull the halves apart. Carefully pry the pit out using the tip of a paring knife, and remove skin.

2. Cut avocado and tomato into wedges, and chop endive crosswise into 2-inch sections (discard base section).

3. Whisk oil and lemon together, and add salt and pepper to taste.

4. Divide salad evenly onto two plates. Drizzle dressing over the top and toss gently to coat.

Serves 2.

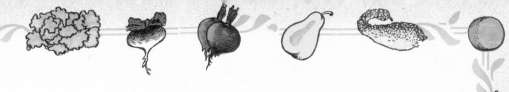

ASIAN CHOPPED SALAD

(Benefits: The variety of veggies in this delicious salad satisfies loads of your daily nutritional goals. The tofu is a great source of protein and calcium.)

Ingredients

3 cups fresh baby spinach

1 cup snow peas, trimmed

1 cup radicchio

$^1/_2$ cup drained sliced water chestnuts

1 $^1/_2$ cups fresh silken tofu, cut in cubes

$^1/_2$ cup daikon (Japanese radish)

$^1/_2$ cup grated carrot

$^1/_4$ cup rice wine vinegar

2 tablespoons canola oil

2 tablespoons soy sauce (low-sodium) or tamari

1 teaspoon sugar

$^1/_2$ cup mushrooms (e.g., white, enoki, grilled portabella)

1. Coarsely chop spinach, snow peas, radicchio, and water chestnuts. Toss in large bowl with tofu, daikon and grated carrot.

2. Whisk vinegar, oil, soy, and sugar together until sugar is dissolved.

3. Drizzle dressing over salad and toss to coat.

4. Top with mushrooms and serve.

Serves 2 to 3.

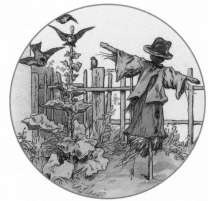

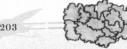

The Shepherd's Wife

William Maxwell

THERE WAS A SHEPHERD'S WIFE in Bohemia who was greatly
saddened when, after twelve years of being married, she still
had no children. Her husband was a quiet man, large and slow-
moving and dependable, and she loved him with all her heart, but
he had no gift for speech, perhaps from spending so much time
with animals, and instead of the prattle of childish voices that she
so longed to hear, the woman was forced to be content with the
ticking of the clock and the sound of the teakettle on the crane,
the singing of wet wood on the hearth. Sometimes her husband
was gone for days at a time, and then the sound of her own foot-
steps grew unbearably loud, and she thought that if only her
husband would come home, so she could hear his heavy sigh when
he sat down and warmed himself before the fire, and the dog's tail
thumping, she wouldn't ask for more—not even the children that
had been denied her.

For every deprivation there is always some gift, and the
shepherd's wife was famous throughout the village for her ability to
make things grow. The windows of her cottage were full of flowering
plants all winter long, and when other women had trouble with
their house plants—the leaves turning yellow and dropping off and

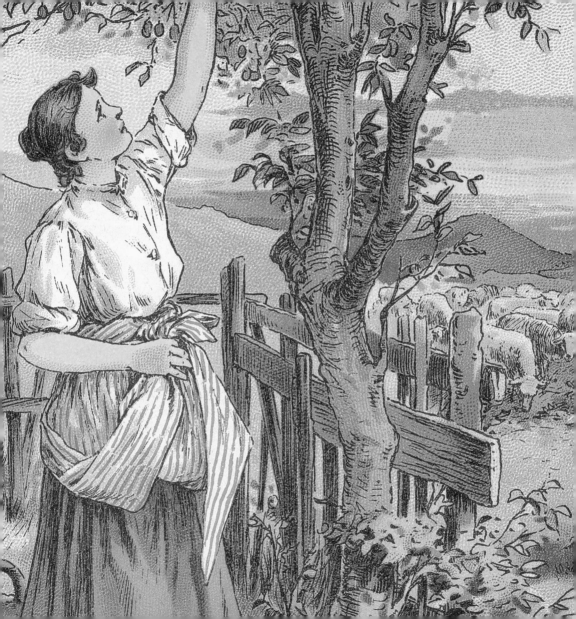

The Shepherd's Wife

no new green coming, or red spider, or white fly, or mealy bug, or aphids—when their favorite plants were, in fact, almost ready to be thrown on the compost heap, they would bring them to the shepherd's wife and say, "Can you do anything with this? It used to have masses of blooms and now look at it!" and the shepherd's wife would make a place for the sick plant on the windowsill on the south side of the kitchen, where the sun poured in all day long through the thick, round glass. A month later she would wrap the plant up carefully against the cold and deliver it to its owner, in full leaf, with new buds forming all over it.

"What ever do you do to make things grow?" the other women asked her. "Do you water them very often, or just every other day, or what is your secret?"

"To make plants grow," the shepherd's wife always said, "you have to look at them every day. If you forget about them or neglect them, they die."

The other women, whose households were blessed with children, never remembered this advice or quite believed in it, and there was even a rumor (for it was a very small place, and no one living there escaped the breath of slander) that the shepherd's wife was a witch.

Actually, there was more to it than she could ever quite bring herself to tell them. After all, they had their little Josephs and Johns and Mary Catherines, and she had only her Christmas cactus,

The Shepherd's Wife

her climbing geraniums, her white rosebush in its big tub, and her pink oleander. So she kept her secret, which was that she not only looked at every plant every day but also talked to them, the way some lonely people talk to animals or to themselves.

"Now," she would say, standing in the front of the Christmas cactus, when the shepherd was out of the house and there was nobody around to hear her, "I know you're slow by nature, but so is my husband, and he has his happy moments and you should have yours. All you need to do is grow a little." Then she would pass on to the pink oleander. "What is *this?*" she would exclaim. "Why are your leaves dry and stiff this morning? Too much sun? Very well, behind the curtain you go until you are feeling better." Then to the white rosebush: "Just because those great geraniums are almost touching the ceiling and crowding everything else out, you needn't think I don't know you are here. Besides, if you will notice, the geranium blossom has no scent...." So she talked to the plants, as if they were children, and, like children, they grew and grew and blossomed over and over again all winter long.

One day, the old midwife who always took care of the birth of children in the village came to the shepherd's wife and, drawing her to the chimney corner where the kettle was boiling for tea, said, "It's time somebody told you—you are with child."

At first the woman wouldn't believe it, although the midwife had never been known to make a mistake in these matters, and when she did believe that it was true, she was still not happy. "I've waited too long," she told herself. "If children had come when I was younger, it would have been very different. Now I don't know what will happen to me. I may die. And if nothing dreadful happens to me, something will certainly happen to my Christmas cactus, my climbing geraniums, my rosebush, and my pink oleander as soon as I take to my bed and cannot look at them and talk to them the way they are used to."

She didn't confide these fears to her husband, not wanting to spoil his happiness, but he knew her moods, and when he saw that in spite of the blessing that had come to them she was still heavy-hearted, he stayed home with her more, and arranged with the other shepherds to mind his flocks for him. Wherever she went about the cottage, scrubbing and cleaning and putting things in order, he watched her, hoping to find out what was on her mind.

Having him around the house so much made her nervous, and when the plants began to drop their leaves and turn yellow because she couldn't bring herself to talk to them in front of anybody, she saw the fulfillment of her worst fears. She became pale, her shoulders drooped, she never spoke of the future, never discussed with her

The Shepherd's Wife

husband what they might name the child, or even whether it was
going to be a boy or a girl. It was as if the child inside her were
somebody else's plant that she could care for with her body but
must not become attached to.

When her time came, the shepherd ran through the snowy
night to the poor hovel that was all the midwife had for a roof
over her head, and brought her hobbling back across the ice and
snow. He put the kettle on the crane and built up a roaring fire
and tried to stop his ears against the sounds that came from the
bedroom—sounds that made his heart stop with terror. He felt a
desperate need to talk to someone, but the midwife was too busy,
coming and going with her hot cloths and her basins of boiling
water, and she would not listen to him. At last he turned to the
plants and told them his fears. Immediately before his eyes the
limp leaves began to straighten, the stems to turn green. He went
on talking to them without perceiving that anything unnatural had
happened. His wife's secret was safe. He was a man, and so it
didn't interest him.

In the terrible course of time, while the shepherd sat with his
head in his hands and cursed the day he was born, the moans in
the next room became screams and cries, and then suddenly there
were two cries instead of one. A little while later, the midwife
appeared with a baby, the smallest that had ever been seen in the

village. She removed the soft woolen scarves it was wrapped in, and showed it to the shepherd, who sprang up with such pride in his heart and such happiness in his face that the newborn babe responded and began to wave its arms feebly.

"You have a daughter," the old midwife said.

"From God," the shepherd said.

"A very small, meachin, puny daughter," the old midwife said scornfully.

"She will be the most beautiful and proud woman that ever lived," the shepherd said. "She will be as beautiful and proud as the forests of Bohemia."

When the old midwife left him to care for the mother and child, he turned again to the plants on the windowsill, and when the sun came up and lighted their leaves, he was still telling them about his newborn daughter.

Day after day the plants grew, but the baby did not, and the mother remained feverish and pale on her bed and did not love her child. When the shepherd knelt beside her and asked how she was feeling, she shook her head and did not say what she thought, which was, I shall never get up out of this bed.

She didn't dare ask about the plants—if they had died one by one, and been thrown out—but one day, after the midwife had gone

The Shepherd's Wife

to assist at the birth of another child, and the man had left the house for a few minutes to see about his sheep, the woman got up out of bed, intending to get back in again as soon as she had satisfied her curiosity. She tottered into the kitchen expecting to see the dry stalks of all her beloved plants, or maybe nothing at all, and what met her eyes was a green bower of blossoms such as she, who was famous throughout the village for her ability to make things grow, had never managed to have. The scent of the flowers was heavy in the low-ceilinged room, and as she stood there, looking at her Christmas cactus, her climbing geraniums, her white rosebush, and her pink oleander, the tight center of her heart opened, petal by petal.

She ran into the bedroom, where the child fretted, and brought it, cradle and all, into the room where the flowers were. "This is my very own daughter," she said. "She's very small, and she cries all the time, but some of you were sickly too, at first, and dropped your leaves, and showed every sign of not flourishing, and now look at you. Dearest heart," she said, pulling back the woolen cover until she could see the shadowy silken skin at the baby's throat. "Now you must grow. You must stop fretting. You must sleep," she said, unbuttoning her dress and helping the tiny pale mouth to find her breast. "You must grow tall and proud and beautiful, like the forests of Bohemia."

Letter to My Unborn Child

Jessie Bernard

4 May 1941

M<small>Y DEAREST,</small>

Eleven weeks from today you will be ready for this outside world. And what a world it is this year! It has been the most beautiful spring I have ever seen. Miss Morris (a faculty colleague) says it is because I have you to look forward to. She says she has noticed a creative look on my face in my appreciation of this spring. And she is right. But also the world itself has been so particularly sweet, aglow with color. The forsythia were yellower and fuller than any I have ever seen. The lilacs were fragrant and feathery. And now the spirea, heavy with their little round blooms, stand like wonderful igloos, a mass of white. I doff my scientific mantle long enough to pretend that Nature is outdoing herself to prepare this earth for you. But also I want to let all this beauty get into my body.

I have so many dreams for you. There are so many virtues I would endow you with if I could. First of all, I would make you tough and strong. And how I have labored at that! I have eaten vitamins and minerals instead of food. Gallons of milk, pounds of

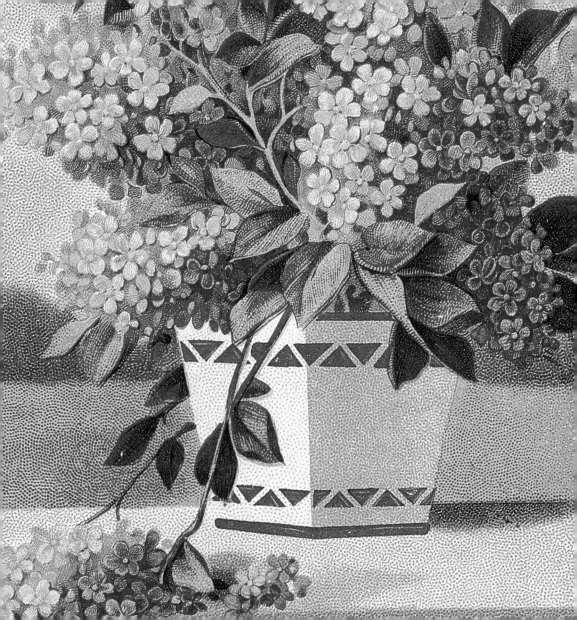

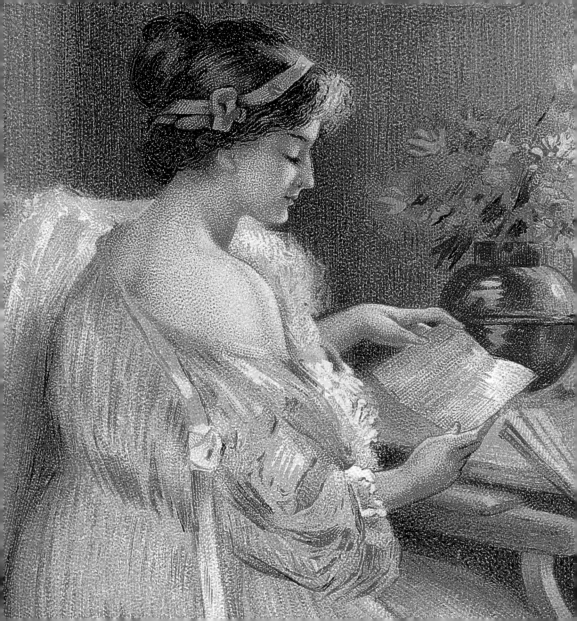

Letter to My Unborn Child

lettuce, dozens of eggs…Hours of sunshine. To make your body a strong one because everything [depends] on that. I would give you resiliency of body so that all the blows and buffets of this world would leave you still unbeaten. I would have you creative. I would have you a creative scientist. But if the shuffling genes have made of you an artist, that will make me happy too. And even if you have no special talent either artistic or scientific, I would still have you creative no matter what you do. To build things, to make things, to create—that is what I covet for you. If you have a strong body and a creative mind you will be happy. I will help in that. Already I can see how parents long to shield their children from disappointments and defeat. But I also know that I cannot re-make life for you. You will suffer. you will have moments of disappointment and defeat. You will have your share of buffeting. I cannot spare you that. But I hope to help you be such a strong, radiant, self-integrated person that you will take all this in your stride, assimilate it, and rise to conquer…

Eleven more weeks. It seems a long time. Until another time, then, my precious one, I say good-bye.

Your eager mother

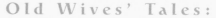

Boy or Girl?

Chances are someone–your mother, your best friend, the helpful clerk at the maternity store–has already pegged it: "Definitely a girl" or, "A boy, hands down." And unless that someone also happens to be your sonogram-ist, your soothsayer probably applied one of many kooky myths.

While wives' tales may have an old logic behind them, few are little more than amusement. But just for fun, we compiled a list of our favorites. Use the quiz below to make your own boy/girl prediction. Read through each set of superstitions and check the first or second column. Tally up each column and– voilà–the higher number is your answer. Whatever the result, you've got a 50-50 chance of being right!

If...

- ...you carry your baby low...
- ...you crave cheese and meat...
- ...you hang your wedding ring over your belly on a strand of your hair and it swings back and forth...
- ...your hands get dried and chapped...
- ...from behind, you aren't noticeably pregnant...
- ...you dream about a knife, a hatchet, or girls...
- ...you rest on your left side...
- ...someone asks you to pick up a key and you do it by the round end...
- ...you hunger for the heels of bread...
- ...you get a hairy belly...
- ...your belly is pointy, like you're birthing a watermelon...
- ...someone drops a penny down your back and it lands on heads...

= it's a boy!

Or if...

- ...you carry your baby high...
- ...you crave sweets...
- ...you hang your wedding ring over your belly on a strand of your hair and it swings in circles...
- ...you hands get softer...
- ... from behind, you are noticeably pregnant...
- ...you dream about spring, parties, or boys...
- ...you rest on your right side...
- ...someone asks you to pick up a key and you do it by the long end...
- ...you prefer the middle of a bread slice...
- ...your face and chest break out...
- ...your belly is round like a basketball...
- ...someone drops a penny down your back and it comes up tails...

= it's a girl!

If need be, here's a surefire tiebreaker:

First, put down this book. Then, imagine a friend saying, "Show me your hands." What would you do? DO IT BEFORE YOU READ BELOW.

Are you holding your hands out? Okay, if they are palms up, you're having a girl. But if they are palms down, you're having a boy, hands down!

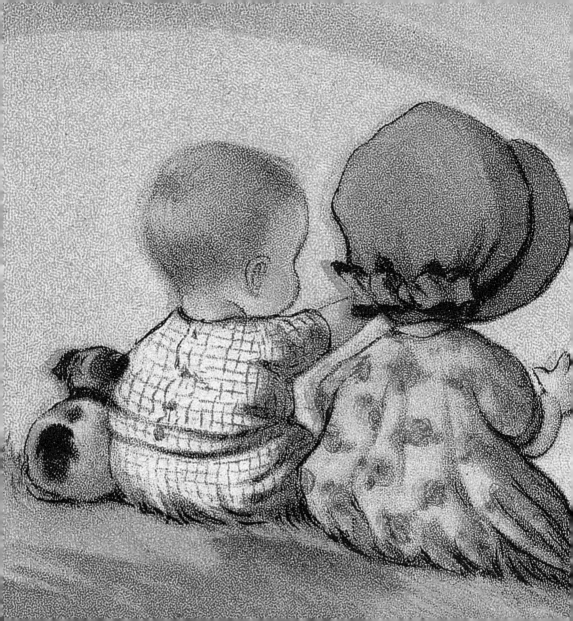

People ask, "Do you want a
boy or a girl?"
The answer is "Yes, of course."

—Anonymous

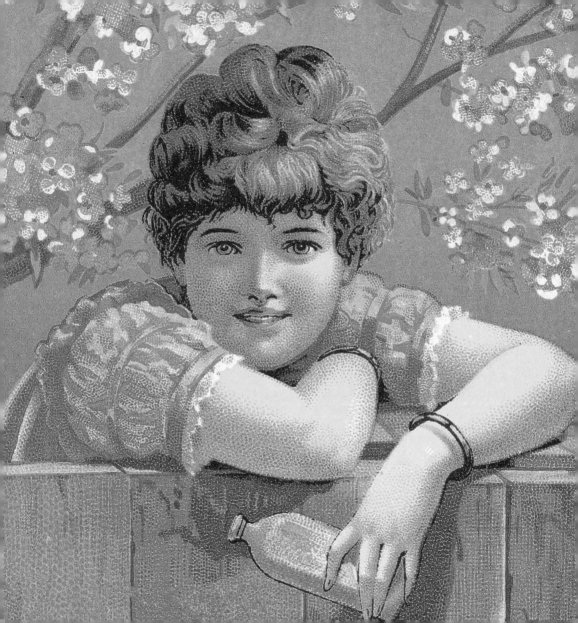

March 19: Starting Late

Bonni Goldberg

Neighbors appear
in sun-warmed air—
on their lawns and backyards
pull weeds, mow grass,
prune back branches, break and turn
the earth,

bend to plant and seed.
Nine months full, as I walk
by with my pendulum belly,
and each face smiles and nods,
I become Spring.

Twilight, porch light,
my husband and I
inhale cut greens, onion, dirt:
like two old monks at the close of day
composting, even from the waste of our lives,
an abundance.

Belly Shadow

This clever activity will allow you and your family to watch the baby grow, much in the same way you saw your own height marked and dated on the kitchen wall or doorjamb during your childhood.

You will need:
Thumbtacks or small nails
Large sheet of poster board
Masking tape
Flashlight

1. Pin, tape, or nail the sheet of poster board to the wall so the top edge is at chest height.

2. Place a strip of tape on the floor, perpendicular to the wall, so that it aligns with the right edge of the poster board.

3. Each month of your pregnancy, stand with your right side to the wall, arms raised, and line your toes up on the tape. Have someone shine a light toward the wall directly at your belly, casting a shadow on the wall.

4. Have a second helper trace the line of the shadow with a felt-tipped pen and write the date on the line. Use different-colored pens for each month. Decorate with drawings, stickers, or stencils. Consider asking friends and family to write little notes to your unborn child on your belly-shadow chart.

5. After the birth, frame the chart and hang in baby's room as a reminder of how he got here and of all the people who loved him on his way into the world.

Belly Cast

No photograph—or even video—could ever capture your pregnant belly as well as this very personal three-dimensional keepsake sculpture. The belly cast will evoke your fondest memories of pregnancy long after it's over and show your child the physical space inside you where she grew.

Make the belly cast in a warm room or outside on a sunny summer day. The plaster gets quite chilly as it sets. Don't try this alone—ask baby's daddy or a good friend to wrap your belly in the plaster strips. To avoid mess, use a drop cloth and have the sculptor wear an apron and surgical gloves (and both take off your jewelry!) You may cast your pregnant body from neck to hips or just your belly by itself.

You will need:

- Drop cloth
- Apron
- Surgical gloves
- Plastic wrap
- Petroleum jelly
- 3–4 rolls plaster gauze casting material cut into 8-inch, 12-inch, and 18-inch strips
- Bowl or pan of warm water
- Premixed plaster of Paris
- Sandpaper
- Gesso
- Craft paint or spray-on acrylic sealer

1. Start by covering your pubic hair with a cloth or plastic wrap.

2. Slather a *generous* amount of petroleum jelly on your skin, completely coating the entire area to be cast. Be careful: The plaster will pull out any hairs it contacts. If your skin is stretched or sensitive, you may want to cover your body with plastic wrap, or wear an old leotard (which you will have to cut off after casting); keep in mind, however, that this will eliminate some of the fine detail, like in your navel and nipples.

3. Sit on a bench or a straight-backed chair for the most natural and rounded shape. Do not lie on your back.

4. Starting with the longest ones, dip each plaster gauze strip into the warm water for a few seconds, then pull it out and, keeping it vertical, get rid of excess water by holding it between two fingers and running them down its length. Have your assistant work quickly to apply the strips, edge to edge, horizontally across the body, covering the entire torso or belly. Smooth the plaster by stroking it flat to the skin. Alternate among different lengths depending on how much surface area you need to cover.

5. Apply a second layer of plaster strips vertically over the first layer, smoothing as you work.

6. Apply a third layer in any direction to strengthen the cast.

7. In 10 to 20 minutes, the plaster will begin to set and the cast will start to pop off the body. Gently pull the edges away from the skin and the sculpture will come off—moving the belly a little can help. (If you are wearing a leotard, your helper must cut it off at the back, leaving the fabric inside the cast. When it dries, trim the excess fabric away.)

8. Allow the "baby belly" to dry for 48 hours; sand any rough edges with a piece of sandpaper.

9. To make a perfectly smooth surface, coat the sculpture with gesso.

10. You can decorate your belly sculpture with paint, or simply coat the belly with acrylic sealer inside and out. *Note: Pregnant women should not be anywhere near this sealant while it's being used. Inhaling the alchohols and fluorocarbons contained in some solvents and sprays can speed up a sensitive heart or cause it to beat irregularly.*

11. Punch two holes, one at each upper corner, for a wire or ribbon to go through. Hang your "baby belly" in the nursery.

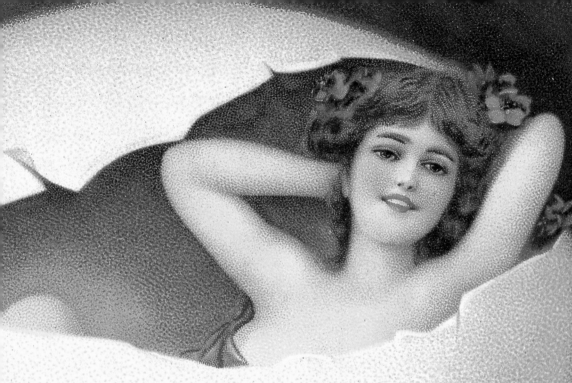

...It's the state of being pregnant,
as if you're weaving a house for
your child out of your own body,
and it takes all your energy,
all your attention.

—Hilma Wolitzer

Your caregiver might call them *striae gravidarum*. Your mother might call them "badges of honor." You might just call them a nuisance. Whatever they're called, stretch marks occur in 50–90 percent of pregnant mothers. In the second half of pregnancy, as your baby grows and your skin is stretched, those unwanted bright red lines may appear on your lower abdomen, thighs, hips, buttocks, breasts, and arms.

When the collagen layer of your skin is continuously stretched, it looses elasticity. Your body responds by sending reinforcements, increasing collagen in the weakened layer and causing stretch marks. Thankfully, the process is not painful. But if your stretching skin tingles or itches, be sure to check our home remedies for skin changes!

So how likely are you to get stretch marks? Your family history plays a role. Did your mom or sister get them? If so, you're a more likely candidate.

Home Remedies: Stretch Marks

Are you gaining weight properly? Rapid, excessive weight gain can make you more prone to stretch marks. Are you eating well and staying hydrated? Healthy, well-hydrated skin stretches better. Did you have stretch marks with previous pregnancies? If you had them before, you'll probably get them again, though usually just temporarily darker, slightly extended versions of your original marks. Your ethnicity is also a contributing factor. Expectant African-American women, for example, are less likely to get stretch marks than lighter-skinned mothers-to-be.

Now, on to the central question: Can your stretch marks be reduced or prevented? Many healthcare professionals insist it's simply a matter of genetics: Some women get them, and others don't. But many still advise that weight management and healthy skin can reduce the severity of stretch marks, and that the daily use of creams can help them fade.

Here are some specific suggestions. See what works for you and try not to obsess! After delivery, stretch marks naturally fade to shallow, often hardly noticeable scars that are lighter in color than the surrounding skin.

Nutrition and Exercise

- Eat a properly balanced diet to help your skin stay healthy.

- Eat ample amounts of protein and foods high in vitamin C for healthy, fast-healing skin.

- Eat foods high in zinc, such as ginger, cheese, and whole grains, which may help prevent stretch marks.

- Drink plenty of fluids; well-hydrated skin stretches better.

Creams and Massage*

- Wear a support bra regularly from the moment you learn you are pregnant.

- Massage abdomen, breasts, hips, and thighs twice daily, as soon as your "bump" becomes obvious, with a good body lotion. Use a cream with evening primrose, vitamin E, or both. As your stomach grows, increase the area you massage.

Consult your caregiver for appropriate massage techniques.

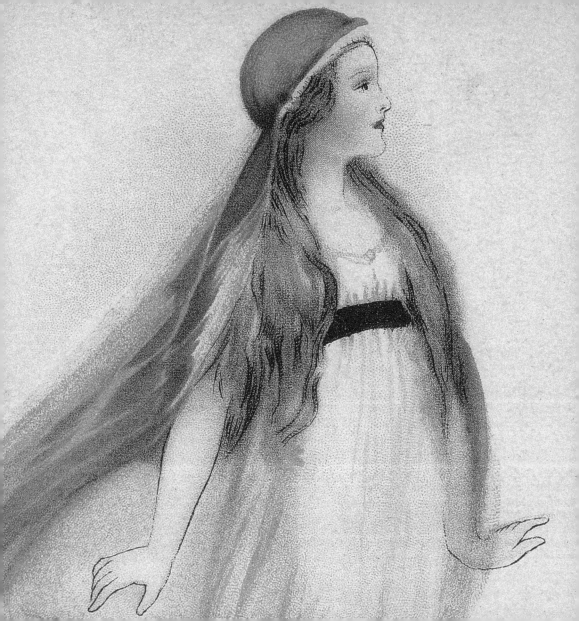

Maternity Fashion Advice

Vicki Iovine

1. Don't Be a Snob; Buy Your Clothes From Any Kind of Store That Has What You Need.

2. At the Very Least, Buy a Bra, Panty Hose, Leggings, Jeans and a Bathing Suit From a Maternity Store.

3. Pick a Style and Stick With It Religiously. This Is Not a Time to Experiment.

4. Always Move Into Bigger Clothes Earlier Rather Than Later; You Will Save Yourself a Lot of Discomfort and, Possibly, Some Embarrassment.

5. Borrow Anything You Can.

6. Never Justify Buying an Expensive Outfit by Telling Yourself You Can Still Wear It After the Baby Is Born. If You Ever Wear That Outfit Again After You Have Gotten Your Figure Back, I Volunteer to *Eat* It.

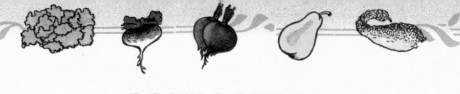

COZY SOUPS

Soup...glorious soup...you and your baby's favorite diet. Soups made with fresh, healthful ingredients can satisfy as many as five of your daily nutritional requirements in a single bowl. They are also a terrific source of fluids. Pairing hearty soups with cheese, bread, and fruit can make for a delicious, well-balanced meal.

BROCCOLI-SPINACH SOUP

(Benefits: The dietary value of this scrumptious soup is off the charts. Broccoli—the most nutritious of the cruciferous vegetables—is packed with vitamins A and C and a broad array of minerals. Spinach is high in folic acid and potassium—two nutrients your baby can't do without!)

Ingredients

6 cups vegetable or chicken stock

10 ounces chopped broccoli, fresh or frozen

10 ounces chopped spinach, fresh or frozen

1 carrot, peeled and sliced

1 celery stalk, sliced

1 medium onion, diced

Freshly ground black pepper to taste

1. Heat stock to boiling and add remaining ingredients. Cover and simmer until tender, about 20 minutes.

2. Cool slightly.

3. Purée soup, a small amount at a time, in a blender or food processor until smooth.

Serves 6.

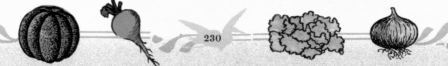

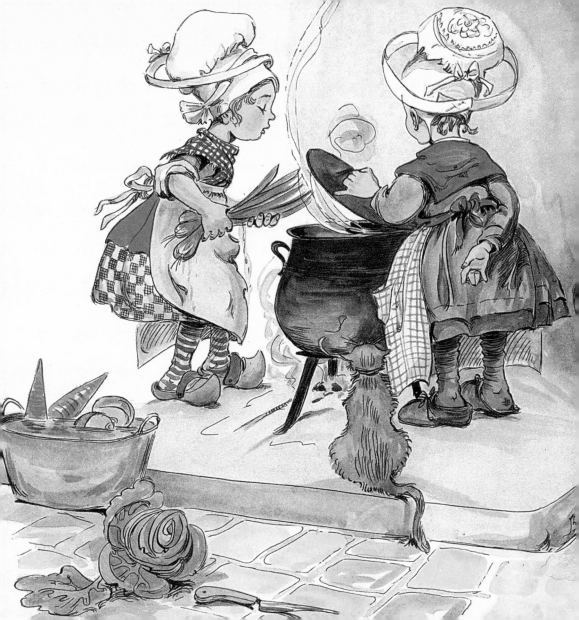

CREAMY CARROT-GINGER SOUP

(Benefits: Dark orange fruits and vegetables tell you that they are packed with vitamins essential for you and your baby's health. Carrots are high in vitamin A, beta-carotene, and fiber.)

Ingredients

6 large carrots, peeled and sliced

2 celery stalks with leaves, sliced

$\frac{1}{4}$ cup crystallized ginger, chopped

7 cups low-fat chicken broth

$\frac{1}{2}$ cup cooked rice

$\frac{1}{2}$ cup whole milk or half-and-half

Kosher salt to taste

1. Add carrots, celery, ginger, and chicken broth to a stockpot. Cover and simmer until tender, about 20 minutes.

2. Add the cooked rice, and allow the mixture to cool.

3. Purée soup, a small amount at a time, in a blender or food processor.

4. Return to heat and add milk. Heat through without boiling, and serve.

Serves 4 to 6.

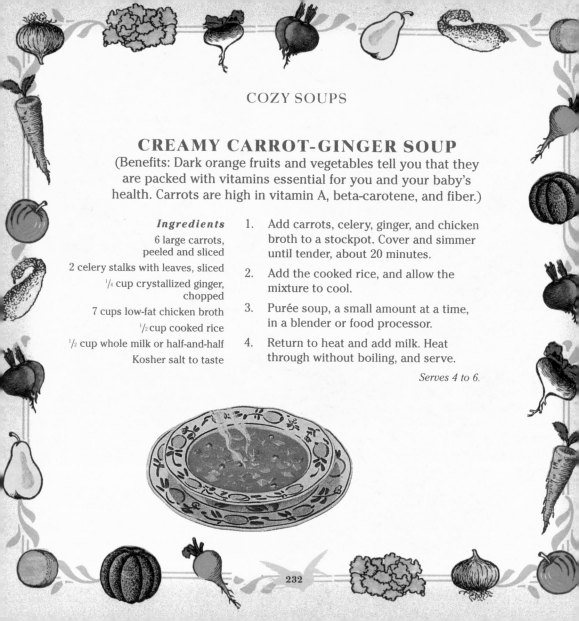

ZESTY BLACK BEAN-AND-RICE SOUP

(Benefits: The bean and rice combination of this easy soup creates a complete protein. But you may wish to add a half pound of browned ground beef or two cups of slightly browned tofu for an extra boost.)

Ingredients

4 cups beef or vegetable broth

2 cups canned black beans, rinsed and drained

1 cup canned pinto beans, rinsed and drained

2 cups sodium-free stewed tomatoes in juice

$^3/_4$ cup instant rice

$^1/_2$ cup chopped onion

1 garlic clove, minced

2 teaspoons vegetable or olive oil

$^1/_3$ cup mild picante sauce or salsa

1 tablespoon chopped fresh oregano (or $^1/_4$ teaspoon dried)

1 teaspoon ground cumin

1. Sauté onion and garlic in oil.

2. Add the remaining ingredients and cook, covered, until rice is tender.

Serves 6.

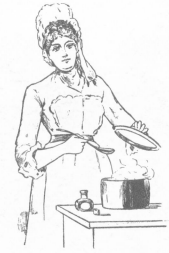

THE NAME GAME

It is one of the most enjoyable tasks of pregnancy—choosing your new baby's name. As you search out the perfect name for your child you are likely to consult many books, friends, and family members for inspiration. Whether you end up naming your baby after a great-grandmother or your favorite poet, sifting through the endless lists of options is part of the fun. So to get you started on your baby-naming journey, we've compiled a selection of some popular baby names in countries around the world. Pick a name with personal meaning, and your son or daughter is sure to grow to love it as much as you do.

AMERICA:		FRANCE:		GERMANY:	
BOYS	GIRLS	BOYS	GIRLS	BOYS	GIRLS
Jacob	Emily	Julien	Amandine	Florian	Katharina
Michael	Hannah	Michel	Chloe	Dieter	Mina
Joshua	Madison	Pierre	Nicolette	Anton	Sophia
Matthew	Samantha	Phillipe	Camille	Maximilian	Katja
Andrew	Ashley	Sebastien	Brigitte	Lucas	Michelle
Joseph	Sarah	Francois	Manon	Jurgen	Inge
Nicholas	Elizabeth	Chantal	Nicolas	Hans	Anna
Anthony	Kayla	Christophe	Lea	Niklas	Hanne
Tyler	Alexis	Killian	Anais	Claus	Sara
Daniel	Abigail	Blaise	Romane	Erich	Franziska

IRELAND:

Boys	Girls
Conor	Chloe
Sean	Ciara
Jack	Sarah
James	Aoife
Adam	Emma
Aaron	Niamh
Dylan	Rachel
David	Megan
Michael	Rebecca
Daniel	Lauren

ENGLAND:

Boys	Girls
Jack	Chloe
Thomas	Emily
James	Megan
Joshua	Olivia
Daniel	Sophie
Matthew	Charlotte
Samuel	Lauren
Joseph	Jessica
Callum	Rebecca
William	Hannah

SWEDEN:

Boys	Girls
Oscar	Emma
Filip	Julia
Simon	Elin
Erik	Hanna
Anton	Amanda
Viktor	Linnea
Alexander	Wilma
William	Matilda
Jonathan	Moa
Emil	Ida

AFRICA:

Boys	Girls
Salim	Asha
Masud	Hadiya
Khalfani	Safiya
Nuru	Zalika
Sadiki	Marjani
Shomari	Ramla
Bakari	Dalila
Sudi	Aziza
Jabari	Rashida
Abasi	Jamila

JAPAN:

Boys	Girls
Daiki	Miku
Takumi	Moe
Kaito	Misaki
Daisuke	Ami
Riku	Rina
Shou	Cho
Akira	Hoshi
Naoko	Takara
Joji	Akina
Tomi	Sachi

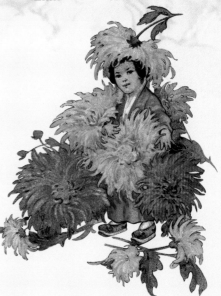

TRADITIONS: *Naming Baby*

A magical task—deciding your new baby's name! The precious name that will mark her place in the world, help form her identity, stay with your child for life... Of course everyone has ideas. And you and your spouse might not agree. Do you name her after a beloved family member? After a heroine from a favorite novel? Or do you pick a name that carries well when you holler out the back door at suppertime? Then there are the other critical tests: making sure you can't spell any embarrassing words with her initials or easily make her name into a schoolyard taunt. All in all, it can be both a fun and daunting process.

How do other cultures choose baby names? In Latvia, it is customary for the godparents to name the infant. In other regions, elders or spiritual leaders provide guidance. As an Inuit mother gives birth, an older female traditionally stands by, calling out possible names. The Inuit believe the baby will be born when she hears the correct name. In Tibet, a high priest (or *lama*) selects and writes down a secret name, which the child will carry in a pouch necklace all her life. Sikh parents randomly open their holy book, the *Guru Granth Sahid*, and read the first letter of the page. A name is then chosen that begins with that letter. Other children are named based on characteristics they develop after birth, as with some African infants, whose physical or personality traits determine their names, such as *Masani*, which means "child who has a gap between the teeth."

The selection of a baby's name is often influenced by religion. Many Roman Catholics and other Christians honor their faith by naming their children

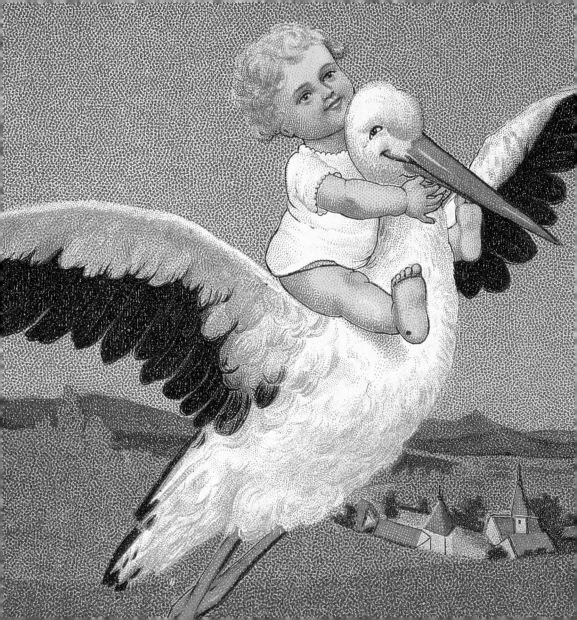

after favorite saints. In biblical times, Jewish families might have used birth circumstances, baby traits, or even nature to help pick a name—e.g., the daughter of a beekeeper might be named *Deborah*, meaning "bee." Many Jews in the Diaspora then started naming children after grandparents, in part to keep track of families and family histories.

Indian children are often given three names: the first is a nickname used by friends and family; the second is used for official purposes, such as school; and the third name is related to the child's individual horoscope, which is prepared using his birth time and specific star alignments. In China, names are thought to greatly influence a child's destiny. Chinese parents carefully select their babies' names according to five traditional concerns. The name must be pleasing to the ear, have a positive meaning (such as one that suggests prosperity or health), be balanced in terms of yin and yang, reflect auspicious math calculations, and contain an element of earth, fire, metal, water, or wood. It's even important *how* the name is written. The number of brush strokes used in a character tells which element that character signifies, and the amount of brush strokes in a name can foretell a child's fortune.

In some cultures, children are named during formal ceremonies. Indians traditionally hold a name-giving ceremony, or *Nam Karna*, on the tenth or eleventh day after childbirth. In northeastern India and Bengal, the naming ceremony is now often performed on the first day a child eats rice, the first day of solid food. According to Jewish tradition, boys are named and circumcised eight days after birth at the bris. An old custom for girls, called *Hollekreisch*, began among Ashkenazi Jews in fifteenth-century Bavaria. During the ceremony, neighborhood children raise the baby's cradle three times, asking "Hollekreisch, Hollekreisch! What shall be this child's name?" Then passages are read from the

Bible, a name is given, and cakes and drinks are served. In Muslim families, the name-giving ceremony, or *Aqiqah*, takes place when the baby is seven days old, after he is gently bathed and his hair is shaved off.

Throughout time, some cultures have given babies false names to mislead evil spirits. In China, unborn babies were often given fake or "milk" names for their own protection. Chinese custom dictated that if babies were called "ugly" or animal names, spirits might pass them over and kidnap other more precious children. According to an ancient Jewish tradition, a name could not only determine a child's fate, it could also thwart the Angel of Death, who might mistakenly overlook a baby named after someone who was already deceased. Korean families, worried about making spirits jealous, traditionally try never to speak positively or cheerfully about a newborn. Children are often called "Dog's Dung," "Stonehead," "Straw Bag," or other unflattering nicknames to protect them from unwanted supernatural attention.

So when it comes time to choose your baby's name, consider some of these age-old traditions. You can ask your elders for naming ideas, and a name-giving ceremony is a beautiful way to introduce your child to the world. Then again, not all traditions are so easily adapted: A false name might protect your child from malevolent spirits, but "Stonehead" will surely fail the schoolyard-taunt test....

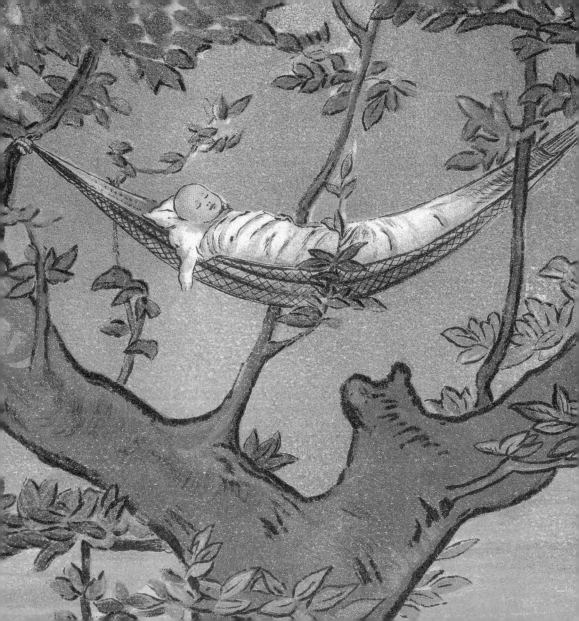

My Baby Has No Name Yet

Kim Nam Jo
Translated by Ko Won

My baby has no name yet;
like a new-born chick or a puppy,
my baby is not named yet.

What numberless texts I examined
at dawn and night and evening over again!
But not one character did I find
which is as lovely as the child.

Starry field of the sky,
or heap of pearls in the depth.
Where can the name be found, how can I?

My baby has no name yet;
like an unnamed bluebird or white flowers
from the farthest land for the first,
I have no name for this baby of ours.

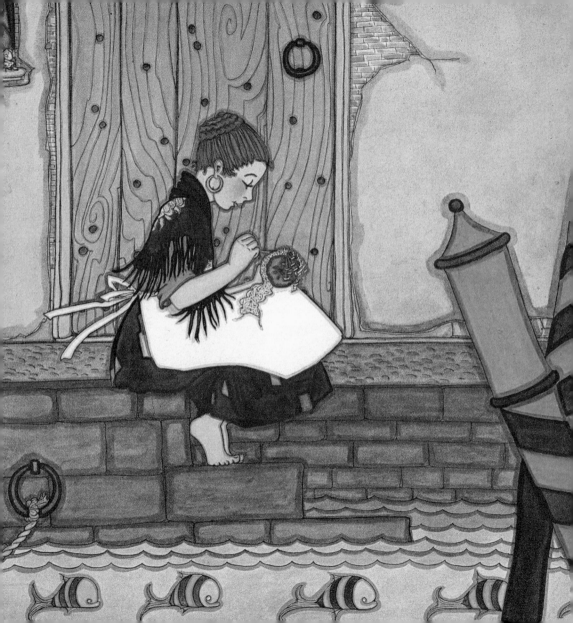

Monogramming 101

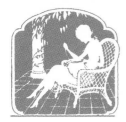

Monogramming the hem of baby's sheets, pillow-cases, blankets, and towels is a wonderful way to personalize baby's bedding and create heirlooms to be treasured for years to come.

Preparing Linens for Monogramming

1. Begin by washing the item to be monogrammed.

2. Select the letters you wish to use from transfer patterns at the fabric/craft store or trace them from the alphabet provided here, using a washable transfer pencil to put the letters directly on your fabric. (For bigger letters, just enlarge our alphabet on a xerox machine and trace.)

3. Traditionally, capital letters are used, with the last-name initial in the center and the first and middle initials, some-what smaller, on either side.

Stitching the Monogram

If your sewing experience is limited, the easiest technique is the satin stitch. This simple stitch makes a smooth, raised letter. Here's how to do it:

1. Use a small embroidery hoop to keep your fabric taught while you stitch.

2. Using two strands of embroidery floss, pull the needle up through the fabric from back to front, beginning at one end of the letter's outline (see *figure A*).

3. Go straight across to the other side of the outline and push the needle through the fabric from front to back. This is your first stitch (see *figure B*).

4. Pull the needle and thread back up through the fabric, next to where your first stitch began.

5. Make another parallel stitch, and keep doing this until you fill the shape of the letter. Be sure that your stitches remain very close together for a more satiny feel and solid appearance (see *figure C*).

6. Keep the reverse stitches as neat as the front. A successful satin stitch should look the same on both sides.

7. When you have filled the letter, tie a neat knot and hide it behind the stitches on the backside.

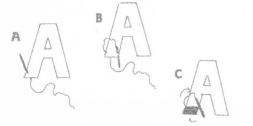

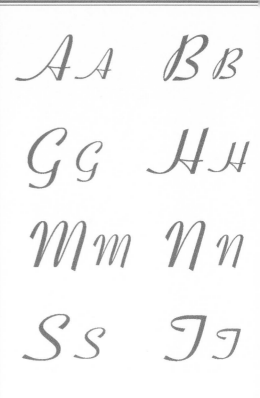

Cc Dd Ee Ff

Ii Jj Kk Ll

Oo Pp Qq Rr

Uu Vv Ww Xx

Yy Zz

Baby Quilt

Stitched by the sturdy hands of women who gathered regularly to sew, quilts are beautifully crafted reminders of a bygone era. Quilting, an American folk-art tradition, provided many an opportunity for family and neighbors to visit over their needlework and collaborate on the beautiful designs. Many quilts were created for hope chests and wedding gifts, or for the arrival of a new baby.

Organizing a traditional quilting bee requires bringing together family and friends on a regular basis—an often difficult task in today's busy world. But by adding a modern twist, you can still make a personalized quilt for your newborn that is the result of a loving and collective effort.

Note: This activity does require some sewing know-how. If your seamstress skills are minimal, however, you can still participate by delegating responsibilities. Follow steps 1 and 2. Then, instead of sewing the quilt yourself, take fabric squares, design instructions, and other materials to a local tailor. He or she should be able to put it together fairly inexpensively. (And no one else has to know it wasn't you!)

You will need:

I yard washable fabric for quilt backing (cotton, flannel, or washable silk)

Spool of thread in color to match fabric

I yard washable solid-color fabric cut into twelve 9″ x 12″ rectangles

24″ x 36″ quilt batting

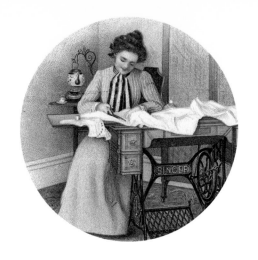

4. Line up the seams and stitch all four rows together, one above the other, to create a rectangular quilt.

5. Cut fabric to size for the back of the quilt and baste a layer of quilt batting to the "wrong" side. With "right" sides facing inward, pin the right side of the backing to the right side of the quilt front. Stitch together along the edges, leaving a 10-inch opening along one side.

1. Give twelve friends and family members each a 9˝ x 12˝ rectangle of fabric to use in your baby's quilt. Ask each contributor to appliqué, embroider, or fabric-paint their swatch in their own design by a certain date.

6. Pull the quilt right side out and close the opening with a slipstitch. Sew the layers together along all the seams between the fabric rectangles.

2. Once all the swatches have been designed and returned, lay them out, in four horizontal rows of three rectangles each, in a pleasing pattern.

3. Stitch the rectangles together. All sewing is with a half-inch seam allowance. Press the seams to one side.

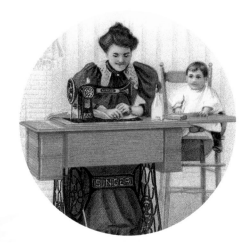

Handkerchief Bonnet

You will need:

12″ x12″ handkerchief

Two 12″ lengths ribbon, ¹/₂″ width

Needle and thread

This easy-to-make heirloom bonnet comes to us from our dear friend Marsha. During Marsha's first pregnancy her mom gave her one of her grandmother's embroidered handkerchiefs and showed her how to make a baby bonnet out of it. Marsha's newborn daughter, Wendy, wore that bonnet the day she came home from the hospital. When she grew up, Marsha snipped the stitches and gave Wendy her great-grandma's hanky to carry on her wedding day. Now Wendy has that handkerchief tucked away to sew into a bonnet again someday for her own baby daughter.

1. Place a 12-inch-square ladies' handkerchief right side down.

2. Sew a gathering stitch along one edge, starting and ending 1 inch from each side. (see *figure A*).

3. Draw the thread together and tightly knot it off.

4. Sew corners together to make gathered circle (see *figure B*).

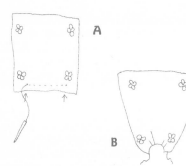

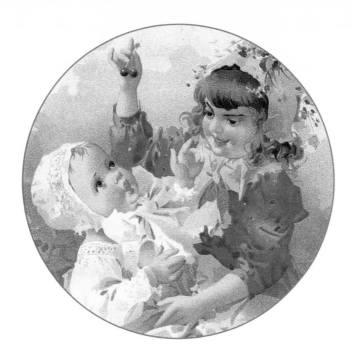

5. Fold the opposite edge over, making a "hem" 4 ¹/₂ inches deep (see *figure C*).

6. Fold the end of a piece of ribbon over about ¹/₂ inch to hide the cut edge. Stitch the folded end of the ribbon to one corner of the hem. Finish by neatly knotting thread on the inside of the bonnet. Repeat on the other corner and your bonnet is complete (see *figure D*).

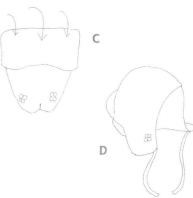

C

D

Childbirth

The time has come. Nine months of planning, preparations, and expectations culminate in this one, magical moment—the birth of your baby! Throughout history pregnant mothers and their caregivers have had varying ideas about how to best anticipate and ease childbirth. And it's not surprising that, along the way, many an Old Wife has also thrown in her two cents' worth.

One favorite belief is that more babies are born during full moons. Some people swear that the gravitational pulls associated with moons and tides can cause Mom's water to break. But even though hospitals *seem* flooded with birthing mothers when the moon is full or at other times of low barometric pressure (during tornados, hurricanes, and snowstorms), studies show there is no documented increase in births.

Another old favorite is that once you've had a cesarean, you'll always need a Caesarean. Though this used to be common procedure, women began having more frequent VBACs (vaginal birth after cesareans) in the 1980s. Nowadays, 50–80 percent of expectant mothers who've had cesareans can have vaginal deliveries.

Other traditional wives' tales are meant to ensure smooth, speedy births. Many cultures have superstitions involving knots and obstacles. East Indian mothers to be are not to tie any knots while they are pregnant. Toumbuluh

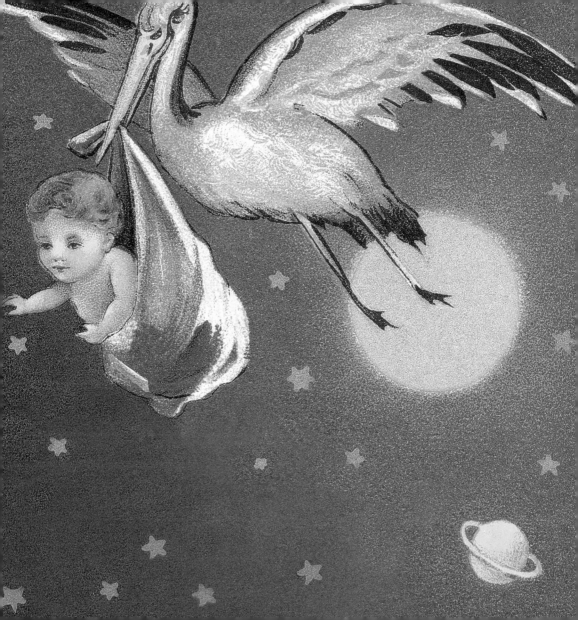

husbands mustn't tie knots or sit cross-legged until their wives give birth. Pregnant Navaho women don't hang out the wash for fear of knotting the baby's umbilical cord.

During labor, the "unknotting" beliefs kick into high gear. To make sure they aren't knotted up inside, women giving birth in Argyllshire, Scotland, are careful not to wear any clothes with knots. On the Island of Sakhalin, in the North Pacific, the laboring woman's husband frees everything inside and outside the house, unlacing shoelaces, taking axes out of logs, and unloading guns. When a woman is in difficult labor in Chittagong, Pakistan, the midwife requests that all bottles be uncorked, all windows and doors be opened, and all animals be freed from leashes and stalls.

Then again, certain obstacles can be beneficial. Some cultures prepare for childbirth by shutting windows and doors and plugging holes to bar the entry of evil spirits. In Sumatra, Indonesia, the midwife might tie a ribbon around the wrist of the woman in labor to prevent her soul from leaving her body. In the Southern Celebes islands, all exits to the house are blocked so the baby's soul doesn't get lost. Also, participants must keep their mouths tightly closed so as not to swallow the infant's spirit. Even the mouths of pets are tied shut!

Still other traditional beliefs involve birthing totems. Expectant mothers of ancient Mexico wore snail-shell charms to help their babies emerge as smoothly as a snail popping its head out of its shell. In France during the 1600s, women in labor kept a "Rose of Jericho" flower and a lit candle beside their bed. The opening flower represented a woman's body at childbirth and the candle timed her labor. Members of the ancient and prestigious Indian Rajput caste "cut" the pain of labor by putting a knife, ploughshare, and sickle under the laboring woman's bed. On the Mediterranean island of Malta, many women hold a statue of Saint Calogero during childbirth. When Japan's Crown Princess Masako went into labor in November of 2001, well-wishers gathered outside the royal hospital holding dogs, traditional Japanese symbols of a safe, painless childbirth.

Of course some Old Wives' tales can now be confirmed by science. One saying asserts that your first child is usually born late. Since approximately 35 percent of babies arrive early and 5 percent arrive right on time, the other 60 percent of babies are born after their due date, making it somewhat more likely that your first baby is late. The Old Wives also like to say that childbirth gets easier with every child. This seems to be true for a majority of women. Labor lasts an average of 14 hours for the first child and 6–7 hours for the second. With each additional birth, labor length may successively decrease by slight amounts. Some say labor is reduced because experienced mothers are less anxious and more self-assured.

Caregivers stress that your health and attitude (as well as the baby's position and size) will play an essential role in determining the length and ease of your labor. With that in mind, eat well, get rest and gentle exercise, and think happy thoughts! And if you still have a "knot" in your stomach, untie the laces of your old shoes in the closet. As long as you're not currently wearing them, what's the harm?

The Blue Jay's Dance

Louise Erdrich

Women's Work

Rocking, breathing, groaning, mouthing circles of distress, laughing, whistling, pounding, wavering, digging, pulling, pushing— labor is the most involuntary work we do. My body gallops to these rhythms. I'm along for the ride, at times in some control and at others dragged along as if foot-caught in a stirrup. I don't have much to do at first but breathe, accept ice chips, make jokes—in fear and pain my family makes jokes, that's how we deal with what we can't change, how we show our courage.

* * *

The first part of labor feels, to me anyway, like dance exercises— slow stretches that become only slightly painful as a muscle is pulled to its limit. After each contraction, the feeling subsides. The contractions move in longer waves, one after another, closer and closer together until a sea of physical sensation washes and then crashes over. In the beginning I breathe in concentration, watching Michael's eyes. I feel myself slip beneath the waves as they roar over, cresting just above my head. I duck every time the

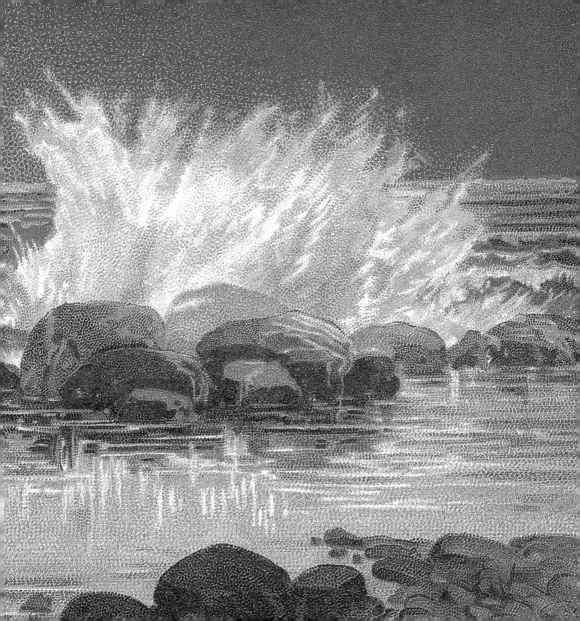

contraction peaks. As the hours pass and one wave builds on another there are times the undertow grabs me. I struggle, slammed to the bottom, unable to gather the force of nerve for the next. Thrown down, I rely on animal fierceness, swim back, surface, breathe, and try to stay open, willing. Staying *open and willing* is difficult. Very often in labor one must fight the instinct to resist pain and instead embrace it, move toward it, work with what hurts the most.

The waves come faster. Charlotte asks me to keep breathing *yes, yes*. To say yes instead of shuddering in refusal. Whether I am standing on the earth or not, whether I am moored to the dock, whether I remember who I am, whether I am mentally prepared, whether I am going to float beneath or ride above, the waves pound in. At shorter intervals, crazy now, electric, in storms, they wash. Sometimes I'm gone. I've poured myself into some deeper fissure below the sea only to be dragged forth, hair streaming. During transition, as the baby is ready to be pushed out into life, the waves are no longer made of water, but neons so brilliant I gasp in shock and flourish my arms, letting the colors explode from my fingertips in banners, in ribbons, in iridescent trails—of pain, it is true, unendurable sometimes, and yet we do endure.

***

The Blue Jay's Dance

Some push once, some don't push at all, some push in pleasure, some not and some, like me, for hours. We wreak havoc, make animal faces, ugly bare-toothed faces, go red, go darker, whiter, stranger, turn to bears. We choke spouses, beat nurses, beg them, beg doctors, weep and focus. It is our work, our body's work that is involved in its own goodness. For, even though it wants at times to lie down and quit, the body is an honest hard-working marvel that gives everything to this one task.

In Praise of My Husband's Hair

A woman is alone in labor, for it is an unfortunate fact that there is nobody else who can have the baby for you. However, this account would be inadequate if I did not speak of the scent of my husband's hair. Besides the cut flowers he sacrifices his lunches to afford, the purchase of bags of licorice, the plumping of pillows, steaming of fish, searching out of chic maternity dresses, taking over of work, listening to complaints and simply worrying, there was my husband's hair.

His hair has always amazed stylists in beauty salons. At his every first appointment they gather their colleagues around Michael's head. He owns glossy and springy hair, of an animal vitality and resilience that seems to me so like his personality. The Black Irish on

The Blue Jay's Dance

Michael's mother's side of the family have changeable hair—his great-grandmother's went from black to gold in old age, Michael's went from golden-brown of childhood to a deepening chestnut that gleams Modoc black from his father under certain lights. When pushing each baby I throw my arm over Michael and lean my full weight. When the desperate part is over, the effort, I turn my face into the hair above his ear. It is as though I am entering a small and temporary refuge. How much I want to be little and unnecessary, to stay there, to leave my struggling body at the entrance.

Leaves on a tree all winter that now, in your hand, crushed, give off a dry, true odor. The brass underside of a door knocker in your fingers and its faint metallic polish. Fresh potter's clay hardening on the wrist of a child. The slow blackening of Lent, timeless and lighted with hunger. All of these things enter into my mind when drawing into my entire face the scent of my husband's hair. When I am most alone and drowning and think I cannot go on, it is breathing into his hair that draws me to the surface and restores my small courage.

Archery

During a time of grief in my father and mother's house, during a period when their adolescent children seemed lighted with a self-destructive fire beyond their control, I found the quote so often used about children written on a scrap of paper in my father's odd and lovely handwriting.

You are the bows from which your children as living arrows are sent forth....Let your bending in the archer's hand be for gladness.

Because my parents for a time practiced archery, I know what it is to try to bend a bow that was too massive for my strength. In the last stages of labor, gathering into each push and bearing the strange power of transition, a woman bends the great ash bow with an unpossessed power. She struggles until her body finds the proper angle, the force, the calm. The fiberglass, the burnished woods, increase in tension and resilience. Each archer feels the despairing fear it cannot be done. But it will, somehow. Walking in the streets or the trails sometimes, now, looking at the women and their children as they pass, I think of them all as women who have labored, who have bent the bow too great for their strength.

At last, with the birth of each daughter, Michael and I experience a certainty of apprehension, a sensation so profound that I feel foggy brained attempting to describe how, in the first moment after birth, the *actual being* of a new person appears.

We touch our baby's essential mystery. The three of us are soul to soul.

Now That I Am Forever with Child

Audre Lorde

How the days went
while you were blooming within me
I remember each upon each—
the swelling changed planes of my body
and how you first fluttered, then jumped
and I thought it was my heart.

How the days wound down
and the turning of winter
I recall, with you growing heavy
against the wind. I thought
now her hands
are formed, and her hair
has started to curl
now her teeth are done
now she sneezes.
Then the seed opened
I bore you one morning just before spring
My head rang like a fiery piston
my legs were towers between which
A new world was passing.

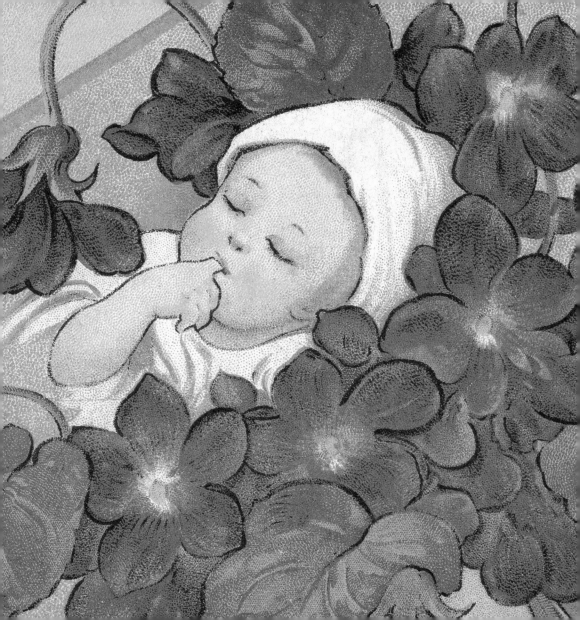

TRADITIONS: *Welcoming Baby*

Your baby will soon be joining your family, joining your community, joining this world. How will you welcome your beloved child? Cultures around the globe greet newborns with celebratory rituals such as name-giving ceremonies, baptisms, and feasts. In many regions, relatives and friends gather to give thanks for a healthy birth and to recognize the boundless potential of a new life, often incorporating religious practices into their festivities. In other parts of the world, babies are more quietly celebrated amongst close family and friends.

Food and drink often have a symbolic purpose as part of a welcoming ceremony. Meat cooked with sugar, for instance, for the Muslim name-giving feast (*Aqiqah*), is said to make a child sweet-tempered. When a Japanese baby is 109 days old, a grain of rice is placed on her tongue to represent acceptance into the community. As a symbol of cleansing, Afghan parents feed babies sugar butter for six days after they're born.

Midwives in Tibet ensure longevity, health, and a lifetime of plentiful food by placing a dab of blessed butter on an infant's nose. When Sikh parents first take their baby to temple and share the *kara parshad* pudding, the baby is given sugared water, or *amrit*. The sugar symbolizes goodness and sweetness, and the water stands for purity. In Ghana, a drop of water, signifying truth, and a drop of alcohol, representing lies, are placed on the baby's tongue. The ritual embodies the hope that the child will always choose to be truthful.

Other cultures use the baby's first bath as an important welcoming occasion. In the region now known as Slovakia, families traditionally would celebrate the first bath by placing tools, coins, salt, sugar, and, in prosperous families, a pen and pencil into the bathwater. Tools and coins represented hopes that the baby would grow into a craftsman or be wealthy. The salt and sugar stood for the wish that the child would someday be decent and well-respected. The pen and pencil symbolized the hope for a good student who would one day become an author or clerk. After the bath, the midwife would hand the child to family members to be kissed and welcomed. People of the Chinese provinces of Kiangsu and Chekiang also celebrated the first bath. A relative would fill two tubs with water: a smaller tub for the baby's head and a bigger tub for the baby's body. Then peanuts and dragons' eyes were dropped into both tubs. The offerings ensured the baby would have a long and successful life.

Some welcoming ceremonies celebrate bonding—connecting the baby to his family and surroundings. For example, Chinese infants are traditionally named and welcomed into the family on their one-month anniversary. On this day, family and friends feast and celebrate throughout the night. Draped around the baby's neck is a gold or silver padlock that symbolically "locks" the infant to this world. Similarly, the Muong in Vietnam ask the newborn's soul to come and eat. A cotton bracelet is used to "link" the baby to her soul.

Some cultures greet newborns with intimate gestures. Members of the Blood Indian Tribe of North America paint the tribe's sign on the infant's face with red ocher and hold the baby up to the sun. The light is meant to follow the baby throughout his life. In Guatemala, a mother may usher her child into the world by approaching trees, streams, and volcanoes and asking them to protect her new baby. Hindu families traditionally bathe the newborn and then write AUM or OM on her tongue using a gold pen dunked in honey. AUM represents Brahma, Shiva, and Vishnu, three prominent Hindu gods. And for Inuit friends and family members, the simple act of shaking the infant's hand is the most welcoming gesture she can receive.

Welcoming your baby into this world can be as simple as an embrace or as elaborate as an organized feast or gathering. However you choose to celebrate the arrival of your little bundle of joy, remember that there is nothing more welcoming than a pair of open arms.

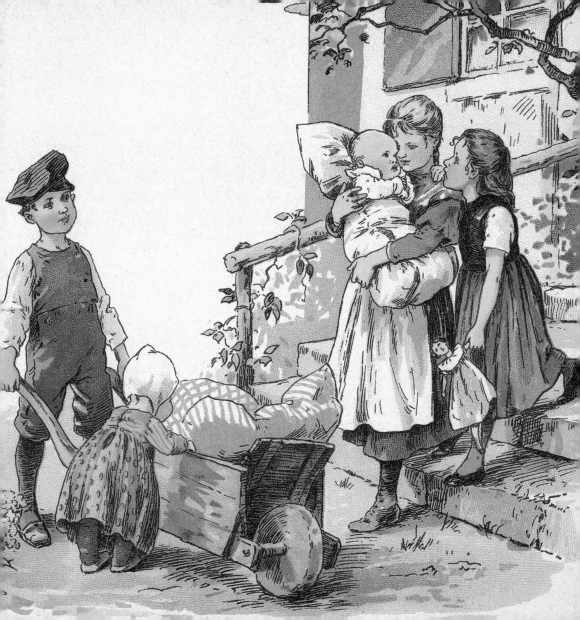

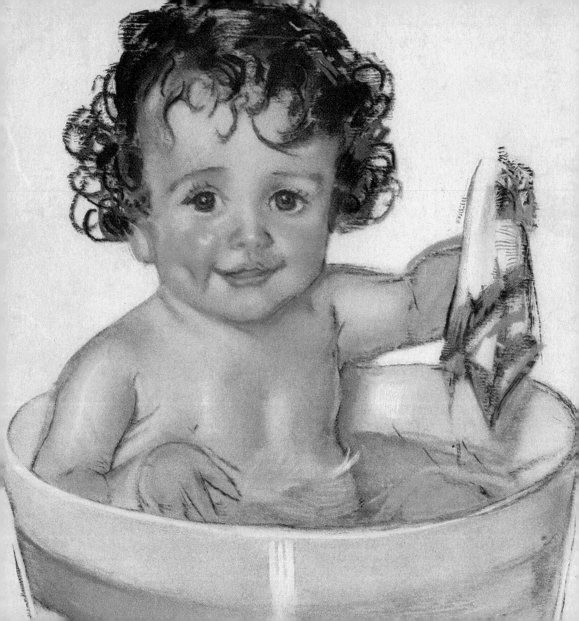

The night you were born,
I ceased being my father's
boy and became my son's
father. That night I began
a new life.

—*Henry Gregor Felsen*

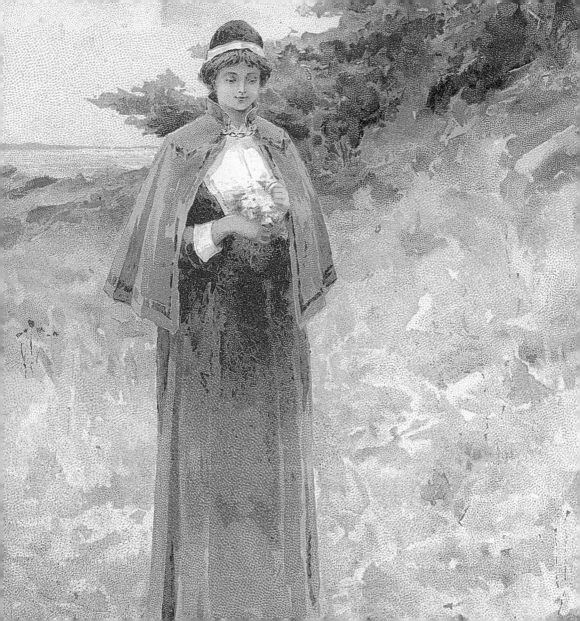

Anna Karenina

Leo Tolstoy
Translated by Joel Carmichael

A T FIVE IN THE MORNING he was awakened by the creak of the
door opening. He jumped up and looked around. Kitty was not
in the bed beside him. But there was a light moving on the other
side of the partition and he heard her walking about.

"What—what is it?" he muttered, half-asleep. "Kitty! What is it?"

"Nothing," she said, coming out from behind the partition with
a candle in her hand. "I didn't feel very well," she said, with a
peculiarly sweet and meaningful smile.

"What—has it begun? Has it begun?" he asked in a frightened
voice. "We'll have to send for—" And he hastily began dressing.

"No, no," she said, smiling and holding him back with her hand.
"I'm sure it's nothing. I only felt a little unwell. It's gone now."

And going over to the bed she put out the candle, stretched out
and quieted down. Though he was suspicious of her stillness, as
through she were holding her breath, and particularly of the
expression of peculiar tenderness and excitement with which on
coming out from behind the partition she had said "Nothing," he
was so sleepy he dozed off at once. It was only later that he

recalled the stillness of her breathing and understood everything that was taking place in her sweet, precious soul as she lay motionless beside him awaiting the greatest event in a woman's life. At seven o'clock he was awakened by the touch of her hand on his shoulder and a soft whisper. She seemed to be hesitating between regret at waking him up and a desire to speak to him.

"Kostya, don't be frightened. It's nothing. But I think…we'd better send for Miss Mary."

She had lighted the candle again, and was sitting on the bed holding the knitting she had been busy with lately.

"Please don't be afraid, it's nothing. I'm not the least bit afraid," she said, seeing his frightened face; she pressed his hand to her breast, then to her lips.

He leaped to his feet, unaware of himself and without taking his eyes off her, put on a dressing gown and stood still, staring at her. He had to go, but he couldn't tear himself away from the sight of her. He would have thought he loved her face and knew every expression it had, every look, but he had never seen her like this. Standing before her as she was now how vile and horrible he seemed to himself when he recalled the grief he had given her the evening before! Her flushed face, framed in the soft curls that had escaped from under her nightcap, was radiant with joy and resolution.

Anna Karenina

Little as there was of affectation and conventionality in Kitty's general character, Levin was nevertheless dazed by what he saw revealed before him now, when suddenly all the wrappings had been removed and the very kernel of her soul shone out through her eyes. And in this simplicity of hers, in this nakedness, she whom he loved was still more apparent than before. She looked at him smilingly; but suddenly her eyebrows twitched, she raised her head and quickly coming over to him she took hold of his hand and pressed all of herself against him, enveloping him in her hot breath. She was in pain; it was as though she were complaining to him of her suffering. And for a moment at first it seemed to him by force of habit that he was to blame. But there was a tenderness in her gaze that told him not only that she did not reproach him but that she loved him for just this suffering. If not I, then who is to blame for it? he thought involuntarily, seeking some culprit to punish for it; but there was no culprit. She suffered, she complained, and she triumphed in this suffering; she rejoiced in it and she loved it. He saw that something splendid was taking place in her soul, but what was it? He could not understand. It was too lofty for his comprehension.

"I've sent for Mama—you go as quickly as you can for Miss Mary...Kostya! No, nothing, it's gone."

She moved away from him and rang. "Well, go on now, Pasha's coming. I'm all right."

And to Levin's amazement he saw her take up again the knitting she had fetched during the night and start working on it again.

While Levin was going out through one door he heard the maid coming in through the other. He paused at the door, and listened to Kitty give detailed instructions to the maid, and with her help start moving the bed herself.

From the moment he had awakened and realized what had happened, Levin had prepared himself to endure everything that lay ahead of him, without reflecting, without anticipating anything, repressing all thought and feeling, determined not to upset his wife but on the contrary to comfort and fortify her courage. Without allowing himself even to think about what was going to happen or how it would end, and judging by the inquiries he had made about how long such things usually lasted, Levin had been mentally prepared to endure and to keep a grip on his heart for some five hours, which it seemed to him he could do. But after this hour another two and three hours passed, then all five that he had set for himself at the most remote limit of endurance, and the situation was still the same; and he still kept on enduring, since there was nothing else to do but endure, every thinking moment that he had come to the ultimate limits of endurance and that at any moment his heart would burst with compassion.

He didn't know whether it was late or early. The candles were all burning low. Suddenly a scream like nothing on earth was heard. He jumped, ran into the bedroom on tiptoe, past Miss Mary and the Princess, and halted at his place by the head of the bed. The screaming had stopped, but now there was a change. What it was he could not see or understand, and he had no desire to. But he could see it by Miss Mary's expression: her face was stern and white, and still just as resolute, though her jaw was trembling a little and her eyes were fixed intently on Kitty. Kitty's burning, agonized sweating face, with a lock of hair sticking to it, was turned toward him trying to catch his eye. Her hands rose, seeking his. Clutching his cold hands with her own sweating ones she began pressing them to her face.

"Don't go, don't go! I'm not afraid, I'm not afraid!" she said quickly. "Mama! Take off my earrings, they're in my way. Are you afraid? Soon now, Miss Mary, soon…"

She spoke rapidly, very rapidly, and tried to smile. But suddenly her face was distorted and she thrust him away.

"No, this is horrible! I'm going to die, die! Go—go!" she cried out, and once again he heard that same unearthly scream.

Levin clutched his head and ran out of the room.

"It's all right! It's all right!" Dolly called out after him.

But no matter what they said he knew that now it was all over. Leaning his head against the doorpost in the next room, he stood there listening to someone shriek and moan in a way he had never heard before, and he knew these sounds were coming from what had once been Kitty. He no longer had any desire for a child. Now he hated that child. he did not even want her to live any more; all he wanted was an end to this horrible suffering.

"Doctor! What is that? What is it? Oh, my God!" he said, grasping the hand of the doctor, who had just come in.

"It's finished," said the doctor. And the doctor's face was so grave as he said this that Levin understood "it's finished" to mean "she's dying."

Beside himself he ran into the bedroom. The first thing he saw was Miss Mary's face. It was even more frowning and severe. Kitty's face was not there. In the place where it had been before there was something strange, because of its look of distortion and the sounds that came from it. He let his head sink on to the wood of the bed; he felt his heart was breaking. The horrible screaming did not stop, it grew still more horrible, and then as though reaching the ultimate limit of horror it suddenly subsided. Levin could not believe his ears, but there would be no doubt of it: the screaming had subsided; a soft stirring was heard, a rustling hurried breathing, and her voice, faltering, alive, tender and happy, said softly: "It's finished."

He lifted his head. Her arms nervelessly outstretched on the quilt, usually lovely and still, she lay there speechless, looking at him, trying to smile but unable to.

And suddenly, from that mysterious, horrible and unearthly world he had been living in for the last twenty-two hours, Levin felt instantaneously transported to the former, everyday world, but now radiant with a new light of such joy that he could not bear it. The taut strings snapped. Sobs and tears of joy he had not in the least anticipated rose up within him with such force that they shook his whole body and for a long time prevented him from speaking.

Falling on his knees by the bed, he held his wife's hand to his lips and kissed it; the hand responded with a feeble movement of the fingers. Meanwhile, there at the foot of the bed, in the skillful hands of Miss Mary there flickered, like the small flame of a night lamp, the life of a human being who had never existed before, and who now,

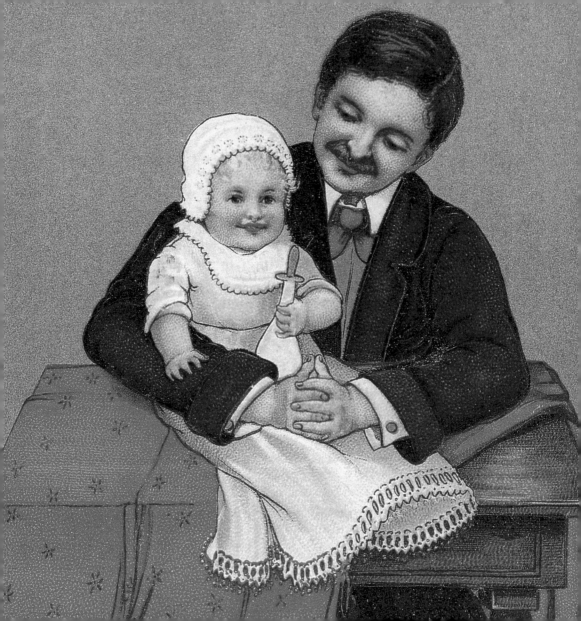

just like others, with the same right and with the same importance for himself, would live and create others in his own image.

"Alive! Alive! And a boy too! Stop worrying!" Levin heard Miss Mary's voice as she slapped the baby's back with a trembling hand.

"Mama, is it true?" said Kitty's voice.

The Princess's only answer was a sob. And amidst the silence, as an irrefutable answer to the mother's question, a voice was now heard in the room that was completely different from all the other voices that had been speaking with such restraint. It was the bold, arrogant, self-centered screech of this new human being who had incomprehensibly appeared from somewhere else.

Before, if Levin had been told that Kitty had died, and that he had died with her, and that the children they had were angels, and that God was there, present before them—he would not have been at all astonished. But now, on his return to the world of reality, he had to make an immense effort of the mind to realize that she was alive and well, and that the creature yelling so desperately was his son. Kitty was alive; the suffering was over; he was unspeakably happy. He understood this, and it made him utterly happy.

The first cry of a newborn
baby in Chicago or Zamboango,
in Amsterdam or Rangoon,
has the same pitch and key,
each saying, "I am! I have
come through! I belong! I am
a member of the Family."

—*Carl Sandburg*

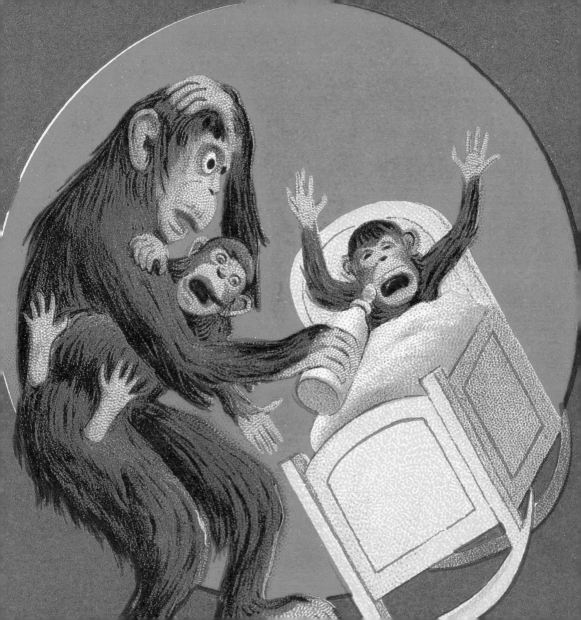

TRADITIONS: *Father's Role*

While the mother's role in childbirth has always been obvious, the father's role—beyond his seminal involvement in conception—varies from culture to culture. Throughout history, men in many areas of the world have opted to steer clear of childbirth. Reasons for their absence include superstitious, religious, and cultural beliefs, as well as just plain squeamishness!

Other fathers are more intimately involved from the earliest days of pregnancy. In many modern cultures, the father to be is encouraged to be an active participant in all aspects of pregnancy, from doing household chores and shopping for the new baby to visiting the obstetrician and attending birthing classes. The pregnant woman often relies on the expectant father to be emotionally supportive, listening to her and understanding her moods. In some cultures, spiritual support goes even further. An old Hawaiian belief purports that the future parents are responsible for the character of their unborn child. Anything they do during pregnancy may influence the baby. Dad, in particular, must be 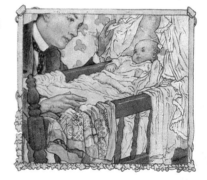 truthful and productive to ensure a virtuous and diligent child. In China, an expectant father traditionally prays at the shrine of Guan Yin, the goddess of childbirth, for the well-being of his wife and child.

So what's Dad to do once Mom goes into labor? In many cultures, childbirth traditionally has been handled exclusively by midwives and other women. Early Native American men were never included in birthing rituals, and instead were relegated to an underground ceremonial hut, called a *kiva*, to pray for their babies' health. In native Brazilian cultures, if a father happened to leave his bows and arrows near his birthing wife the weapons might become cursed and useless. Fathers belonging to the Ik tribes of Uganda were forbidden to enter the house where their child was born until at least a week after delivery.

Even where fathers are expected to make themselves scarce during delivery, many are required to perform valuable behind-the-scenes roles. According to an old Irish tradition, a father can give energy to his laboring wife by having her wear his watch or vest. If a Kenyan Gusii woman has trouble, a midwife might ask the father to gather chinsaga roots for the pregnant woman to chew. Chinsaga juices are said to help coax out the "stuck" child.

An old tradition of *couvade*, which reputedly stems from the Latin word *cubare*, meaning "to lie down," (or possibly the French word *couver*, meaning "to sit on or hatch") requires the father to imitate his pregnant wife. Whether it's clothes swapping, role reversal, or sympathetic labor pains, *couvade* allows the father to share his wife's trials, participate in the birth, and divert evil spirits. This transference ritual is still performed in parts of Africa, India, Malaysia, Siberia, and South America. In rural southern India, men were known to dress in their wives' saris and writhe in mock pain until the labor was over.

Immediately after birth, Bakairi fathers in central Brazil rock newborns in their hammocks while mothers go back to work. The new father is then expected to refrain from eating meat and adhere to a strict diet of bread dipped in water until his infant's bellybutton heals.

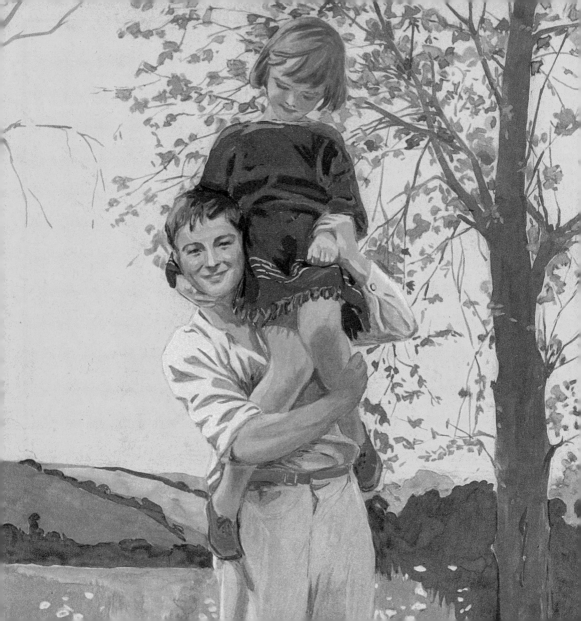

Other traditions seem to have developed as a way to keep the anxious father busy. One example is an old custom from the Irish countryside, where fathers were required to draw bucket after bucket of water until the baby was born and both mother and father were exhausted.

In some cultures, the father is expected to be more intimately involved in childbirth. Amish fathers attend the birth of their children, and many Mennonite mothers want only their husbands to be present. It is the sacred duty of a Tibetan father to attend his child's birth and welcome him or her. Men of the Yucatán are present during their children's births so they can witness "how a woman suffers." And among Himalayan Sherpa families, fathers massage and comfort their wives during labor and then greet visitors coming to see the newborn, ensuring that the new mothers are not overly stressed by social responsibilities.

Once the baby is born, fathers often take on new roles, protecting, providing for, and nurturing their children. Early on, a father from a Roma tribe participates in a ritual to acknowledge his paternity. Mbuti fathers from the Congo fortify and protect both their wives and babies by spritzing them with juice from sacred vines. Muslim fathers, expected to protect and provide hope for their children, put a small piece of a date in their newborn's mouth to symbolize the sweetness of life.

Talk to your partner and discuss his involvement in the birthing process and child rearing in general. Do you plan to divide your parental responsibilities as they do in Malta, where Dad does little more than give out orders? Perhaps your husband would enjoy a northern Japanese custom whereby fathers process their new responsibilities and honorable position by embarking on a 12-day contemplative retreat. Or do you want your household to resemble a Balinese home, where the father spends more time caring for the children than the mother does? Now *that's* worth looking into....

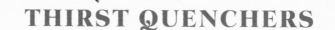

THIRST QUENCHERS

Did you know you and your baby need the equivalent of at least eight glasses of water daily? That's no easy task! Although water is best, there are plenty of ways to spice up your beverage list and help you get some of the nutrients you and your baby need. Some simple options include low-fat or skim milk, 100 percent fruit juice, and low-sodium vegetable juice. Low-sodium soups and juicy fruits and vegetables (such as grapefruit, melon, and lettuce) can also help you get the fluids you require. (Choose fresh fruits and vegetables over canned or frozen whenever possible and avoid all caffeinated drinks, like soda and coffee.) And who says you can't have a festive cocktail now and then? Many virgin drinks and smoothies are so good you won't even miss the alcohol!

BREAKFAST IN A BLENDER
(Benefits: This quick-to-prepare healthful drink is practically a meal in itself as it contains ingredients from three of the four major food groups.)

Ingredients

1 ripe banana
1 peach or nectarine
½ cup low-fat milk
or yoghurt
1 teaspoon honey
1 tablespoon natural
bran or oats

1. Peel fruit, cut up, and place in a blender.

2. Add all other ingredients and blend until smooth.

3. Try adding frozen berries, an apple, or a mango in place of the peach or nectarine. Substituting ½ cup orange juice for the honey will yield a lighter consistency.

Serves 1 to 2.

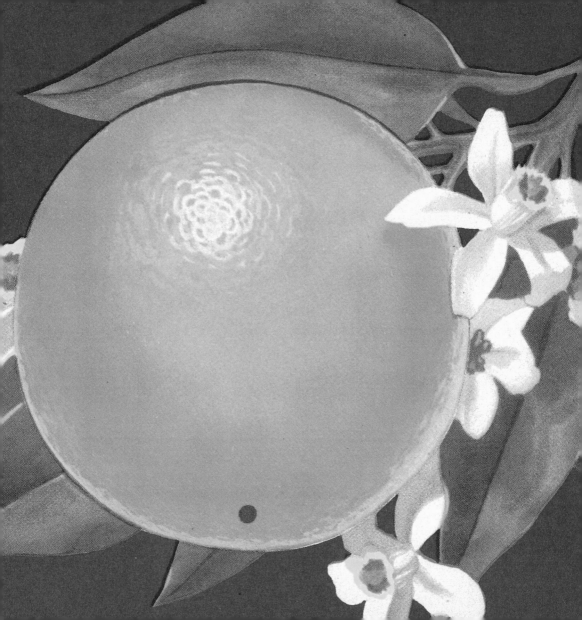

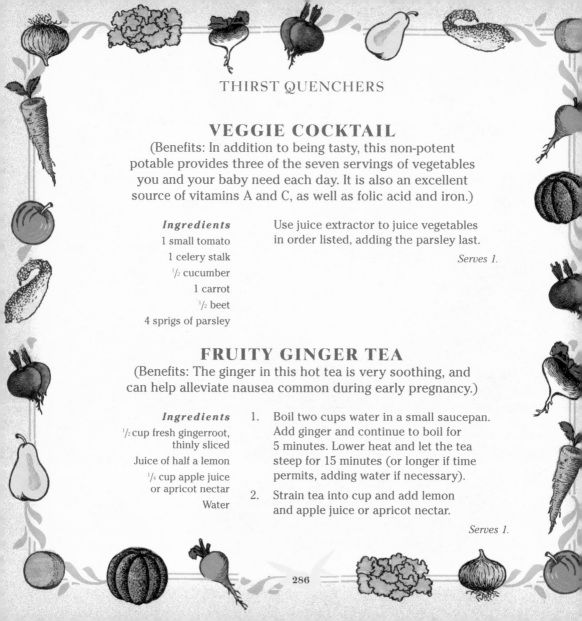

THIRST QUENCHERS

VEGGIE COCKTAIL

(Benefits: In addition to being tasty, this non-potent
potable provides three of the seven servings of vegetables
you and your baby need each day. It is also an excellent
source of vitamins A and C, as well as folic acid and iron.)

Ingredients

1 small tomato
1 celery stalk
$^1/_2$ cucumber
1 carrot
$^1/_2$ beet
4 sprigs of parsley

Use juice extractor to juice vegetables
in order listed, adding the parsley last.

Serves 1.

FRUITY GINGER TEA

(Benefits: The ginger in this hot tea is very soothing, and
can help alleviate nausea common during early pregnancy.)

Ingredients

$^1/_2$ cup fresh gingerroot,
thinly sliced
Juice of half a lemon
$^1/_4$ cup apple juice
or apricot nectar
Water

1. Boil two cups water in a small saucepan.
    Add ginger and continue to boil for
    5 minutes. Lower heat and let the tea
    steep for 15 minutes (or longer if time
    permits, adding water if necessary).

2. Strain tea into cup and add lemon
    and apple juice or apricot nectar.

Serves 1.

CRANBERRY ZINGER

(Benefits: This refreshment is a real boost
to the immune system. Cranberry juice and
cranberries ward off infection, and cranberries
and oranges are loaded with vitamin C.)

Ingredients

1 ¼ cups fresh frozen
orange segments

1 ½ cups 100% cranberry juice

½ cup sorbet (raspberry,
blood orange, or mango)

½ cup fresh frozen cranberries

1. Prepare orange segments by removing membranes prior to freezing.

2. Combine cranberry juice and sorbet in a blender.

3. Add orange segments and cranberries, and blend until smooth.

4. If fresh cranberries are unavailable, use fresh frozen blueberries. For a creamier concoction, use low-fat frozen yoghurt in place of sorbet.

Serves 2.

The Mother Connection

Hope Edelman

IT RAINED the day of my grandmother's funeral, a fine drizzle that
clung to our dark coats like a silver veil. She died this past
December, a few weeks short of her ninetieth birthday. We buried
her in the family plot just behind my mother, who died at forty-two.
The official documents listed my grandmother's cause of death as
acute respiratory and coronary failure, backed up by advanced
breast cancer—an absolute calamity of the chest—but I believe
otherwise: despite all her ailments, she died of loneliness and quite
possibly a broken heart. She kept asking for my mother until the
very end.

The bonds between mothers and daughters have always been
tight in my family—too tight, most of us have complained. It's as if
the women believe that the harder they cling, the more they can
protect. If only that were true. Our stories are marked by departure
and longings, by frustration and despair. My great-grandmother Ida,
leaving Russia at 36 with three children, saying goodbye to the
mother she would never see again. My grandmother Faye, a stub-
born, willful woman with a love so enduring and irrational that it

The Mother Connection

often drove my mother to slam down the telephone or retreat into her bedroom to scream at the walls. My own mother, whose early death from breast cancer left behind two angry teenage daughters and a mother who walked around for months refusing to accept— was never able to accept—the truth.

In the full Bonwit Teller shopping bags my grandmother used to carry wherever she went, she kept a framed photograph of her mother, a serious woman in a dark print dress, who died before I was born. I used to laugh at her for this, teasing her for dragging around a picture of an old woman in the bottom of a tattered paper bag. My mother would hush me, telling me to leave Grandma alone. Only later did I realize the poignancy of this act, how important those bags were to my grandmother's feelings of safety and well-being, and how the image of her mother must have provided the same; how my mother understood this and how by gently quieting her daughter she showed loyalty to an aging mother who at other times nearly drove her mad.

I treasure these memories now, along with the stories these women told me about their lives. As we sat around the kitchen table or took long drives in the car, they handed down women's culture, replete with all its tales of hardship and triumph, loss and rebirth. My grandmother spoke of her mother's ability to stretch a

The Mother Connection

piece of meat far enough to feed seven, and about how she herself studied to become a lawyer only to find she didn't have enough money for the exam fee. My mother told stories about maturing faster than her peers, about how her mother hadn't prepared her for menstruation and how she swore, at age nine, that she would tell her daughter in advance. (She did, when I was eight.)

But now there is no one left who can verify my memories of these women, who heard the exact stories they told me, or can add to them, or tell me which details I've got wrong. At thirty-two, I'm the only woman left in my maternal line, and few things I've encountered have made me feel quite so alone.

I was acutely aware of this as I stood at my grandmother's grave in the gentle rain. Damn it! I wanted to cry out. The last one gone! I understood that I represented a symbolic end point, but I

The Mother Connection

did not yet realize I could represent a beginning, too. So it is
perhaps not all that surprising that when I learned I was pregnant,
less than two months after the funeral, I received the news with
uncharacteristic calm. It was a statistical fluke, one of those birth-
control failures that pull effective rates down into the ninety-odd
percentiles, or so the gynecologist said. I didn't disagree. In the
frenzy that followed—planning a wedding, buying a house, and all
those doctor's visits—there wasn't much time to sit and reflect.
Which is probably why I didn't notice for months that this year I'm
bridging the gap between death and birth. I've lost all my mothers,
but I'm in the process of becoming one, and it's a sweet and healing
continuity that added an unexpectedly profound twist to Mother's
Day this year.

I cried when the ultrasound technician told me the baby is a
girl. How will I protect her? How will I accept that I can't? Each time
I feel one of her kicks, already signaling her independence, I feel a
blend of joy and wonder and fear and grief unlike anything I've
known before. And this is what I think: maybe this child wasn't
an accident after all. Maybe in a family where the love between
mothers and daughters was always so unquestioned and absolute,
a vacuum can't exist for long. Maybe, just maybe, when the last
mother dies, a new one must be born.

Metaphors

Sylvia Plath

I'm a riddle in nine syllables,
An elephant, a ponderous house,
A melon strolling on two tendrils.
O red fruit, ivory, fine timbers!
This loaf's big with its yeasty rising.
Money's new-minted in this fat purse.
I'm a means, a stage, a cow in calf.
I've eaten a bag of green apples,
Boarded the train there's no getting off.

20 March 1959

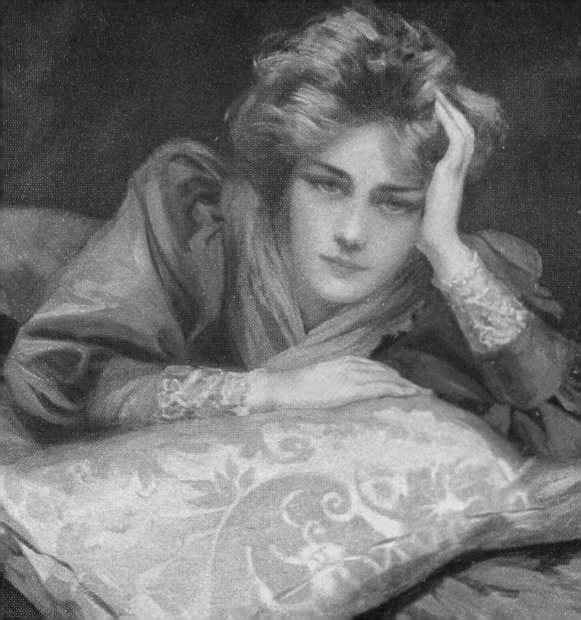

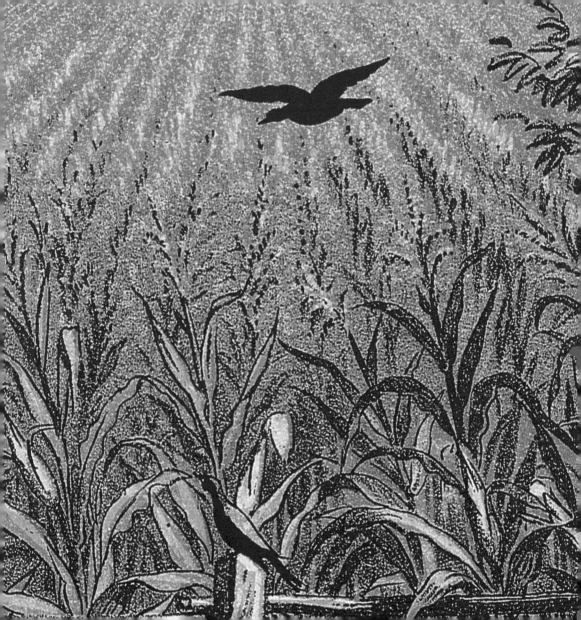

The Good Earth

Pearl S. Buck

SHE WOULD HAVE NO one with her when the hour came. It came one night, early, when the sun was scarcely set. She was working beside him in the harvest field. The wheat had borne and been cut and the field flooded and the young rice set, and now the rice bore harvest, and the ears were ripe and full after the summer rains and the warm ripening sun of early autumn. Together they cut the sheaves all day, bending and cutting with short-handled scythes. She had stooped stiffly, because of the burden she bore, and she moved more slowly than he, so that they cut unevenly, his row ahead, and hers behind. She began to cut more and more slowly as noon wore on to afternoon and evening, and he turned to look at her with impatience. She stopped and stood up then, her scythe dropped. On her face was a new sweat, the sweat of a new agony.

"It is come," she said. "I will go into the house. Do not come into the room until I call. Only bring me a newly peeled reed, and slit it, that I may cut the child's life from mine."

She went across the fields toward the house as though there were nothing to come, and after he had watched her he went to the

The Good Earth

edge of the pond in the outer field and chose a slim green reed and peeled it carefully and slit it on the edge of his scythe. The quick autumn darkness was falling then and he shouldered his scythe and went home.

When he reached the house he found his supper hot on the table and the old man eating. She had stopped in her labor to prepare them food! He said to himself that she was a woman such as is not commonly found. Then he went to the door of their room and he called out,

"Here is the reed!"

He waited, expecting that she would call out to him to bring it in to her. But she did not. She came to the door and through the crack her hand reached out and took the reed. She said no word, but he heard her panting as an animal pants which has run for a long way.

The old man looked up from his bowl to say,

"Eat, or all will be cold." And then he said, "Do not trouble yourself yet—it will be a long time. I remember well when the first was born to me it was dawn before it was over. Ah me, to think that out of all the children I begot and your mother bore, one after the other—a score or so—I forget—only you have lived! You see why a woman must bear and bear." And then he said again, as though he had just thought of it newly, "By this time tomorrow I may be grandfather to a man child!" He began to laugh suddenly and he stopped his eating and sat chuckling for a long time in the dusk of the room.

But Wang Lung stood listening at the door to those heavy animal pants. A smell of hot blood came through the crack, a sickening smell that frightened him. The panting of the woman within became quick and loud, like whispered screams, but she made no sound aloud. When he could bear no more and was about to break into the room, a thin, fierce cry came out and he forgot everything.

"Is it a man?" he cried importunately, forgetting the woman. The thin cry burst out again, wiry, insistent. "Is it a man?" he cried again, "tell me at least this—is it a man?"

And the voice of the woman answered as faintly as an echo, "A man!"

He went and sat down at the table then. How quick it had all been! The food was long cold and the old man was asleep on his bench, but how quick it had all been! He shook the old man's shoulder.

"It is a man child!" he called triumphantly. "You are grandfather and I am father!"

The old man woke suddenly and began to laugh as he had been laughing when he fell asleep.

The Good Earth

"Yes—yes—of course," he cackled, "a grandfather—a grandfather" and he rose and went to his bed, still laughing.

Wang Lung took up the bowl of cold rice and began to eat. He was very hungry all at once and he could not get the food into his mouth quickly enough. In the room he could hear the woman dragging herself about and the cry of the child was incessant and piercing.

"I suppose we shall have no more peace in this house now," he said to himself proudly.

When he had eaten all that he wished he went to the door again and she called to him to come in and he went in. The odor of spilt blood still hung hot upon the air, but there was no trace of it except in the wooden tub. But into this she had poured water and had pushed it under the bed so that he could hardly see it. The red candle was lit and she was lying neatly covered upon the bed. Beside her, wrapped in a pair of his old trousers, as the custom was in this part, lay his son.

He went up and for the moment there were no words in his mouth. His heart crowded up into his breast and he leaned over the child to look at it. It had a round wrinkled face that looked very dark and upon its head the hair was long and damp and black. It had ceased crying and lay with its eyes tightly shut.

The Good Earth

He looked at his wife and she looked back at him. Her hair was still wet with her agony and her narrow eyes were sunken. Beyond this, she was as she always was. But to him she was touching, lying there. His heart rushed out to these two and he said, not knowing what else there was that could be said,

"Tomorrow I will go into the city and buy a pound of red sugar and stir it into boiling water for you to drink."

And then looking at the child again, this burst forth from him suddenly as though he had just thought of it, "We shall have to buy a good basketful of eggs and dye them all red for the village. Thus will everyone know I have a son!"

***

And then, almost before one could realize anything, the woman was back in the fields beside him. The harvests were past, and the grain they beat out upon the threshing floor which was also the dooryard to the house. They beat it out with flails, he and the woman

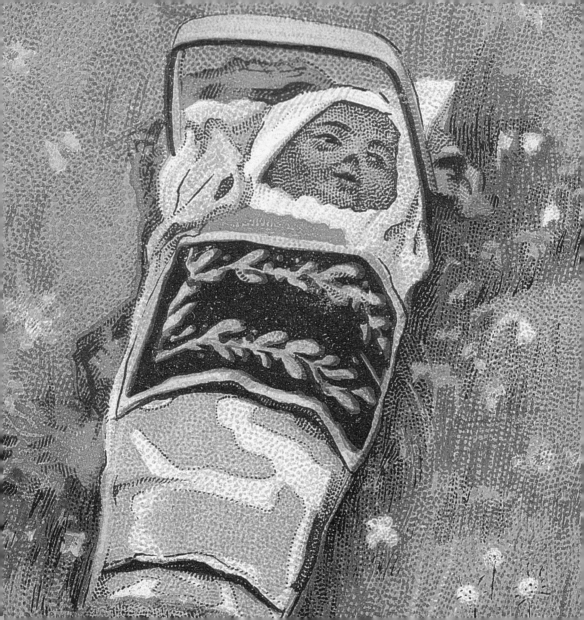

together. And when the grain was flailed they winnowed it, casting it up from great flat bamboo baskets into the wind and catching the good grain as it fell, and the chaff blew away in a cloud with the wind. Then there were the fields to plant for winter wheat again, and when he had yoked the ox and ploughed the land the woman followed behind with her hoe and broke the clods in the furrows.

She worked all day now and the child lay on an old torn quilt on the ground, asleep. When it cried the woman stopped and uncovered her bosom to the child's mouth, sitting flat upon the ground, and the sun beat down upon them both, the reluctant sun of late autumn that will not let go the warmth of summer until the cold of the coming winter forces it. The woman and the child were as brown as the soil and they sat there like figures made of earth. There was the dust of the fields upon the woman's hair and upon the child's soft black head.

But out of the woman's great brown breast the milk gushed forth for the child, milk as white as snow, and when the child suckled at one breast it flowed like a fountain from the other, and she let it flow. There was more than enough for the child, greedy though he was, life enough for many children, and she let it flow out carelessly, conscious of her abundance. There was always more and more.

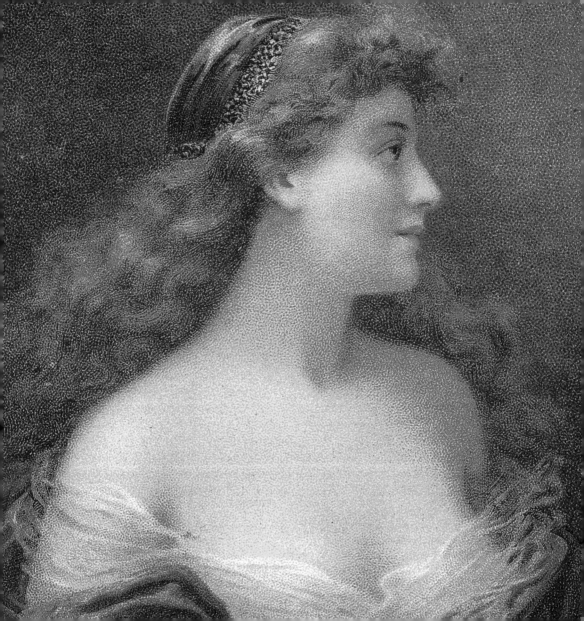

I t's natural—and should be easier than falling off a log, right? Well, while breast-feeding is a healthy and beautiful bonding process, it isn't always stress-free.

After the birth of your baby, your breasts have important work to do. So give your body the care it deserves. Buy comfy, quality, cotton maternity bras. Wear a clean bra every day, changing your breast pads whenever they get wet and using new pads after nursing. Shower or

Home Remedies:
Breast-Feeding

otherwise clean your breasts once a day with cotton balls and water, then pat them dry. (Soap strips your skin of protective, moisturizing oils and covers your natural scent—a scent your baby will recognize.)

There are a few red flags which should cause you to contact your caregiver or lactation expert. Get help if you have a fever or if any of the following conditions last more than twenty-four hours: you are having trouble feeding your baby; your breasts are engorged; you think you have a breast infection—warning signs include hot, reddish skin, severe swelling, hardened tissue, acute soreness, and flu-like symptoms such as fever, aching, and shivering.

But for more common breast-feeding problems, such as engorgement, clogged ducts, or sore nipples, here are some soothing home remedies!

Your Cup Runneth Over

In the days after giving birth, if you skip a feeding or don't routinely empty your breasts, they can become engorged (overfilled). Engorged breasts feel warm, hard, and painfully swollen. While clogged ducts or infections often affect one breast, engorgement typically occurs in both. Address the problem promptly, not only because it's painful, but also because it may cause your body to stop producing milk prematurely. If your breasts become overfilled, use the following tips to ease the pressure, and take heart knowing that, though it may return, the discomfort of engorgement generally disappears after a day or two.

- Relax and take a warm bath or shower.

- Place soothing, heated towels over your breasts to help coax the milk forth.

- Give frequent feedings. If the baby has difficulty latching on, its time to get some expert advice.

- Place cabbage leaves inside your bra with holes cut out for your nipples. Apply for twenty minutes at a time. (Another European tradition suggests using cold rhubarb leaves instead of cabbage. This is supposed to work especially well during the first days of nursing.)

A Clog in the Pipe

During the first few weeks of breast-feeding, some mothers' milk ducts get clogged. Blockages can be caused by pressure from a tight bra, engorged breasts that have been improperly drained, dried milk stopping up a nipple, sleeping on your stomach, poor feeding from the baby, or just plain fatigue. Unlike engorgement, the condition normally occurs in only one breast. Check your entire breast for an area that is uncomfortably swollen. Symptoms may include lumpy red skin and small white spots on your breast. Serious swelling or infections should be examined by your caregiver immediately. For normal blockages, some home remedies include:

- Try to fully empty your breast while nursing and squeeze or pump out any excess milk (keeping in mind that you are *always* making more milk).

- Make sure your nipple isn't clogged with dried milk. If you notice a blockage, first boil some water and let it cool. Then dunk a sterile cotton ball in the water and clean the area. Follow with a hot compress.

- Help unclog ducts by bathing in warm water or swabbing your breasts with a soft cloth dipped in warm water.

- To prevent recurring blockages, make sure your bra fits well and isn't too tight, especially across the upper edges. Consider going to a lactation consultant for an expert fitting.

Ouch, That Hurts!

For the first few days of nursing, your nipples may feel somewhat tender for a minute or two after your baby "latches on." If your discomfort lasts longer or worsens, you may need to pay special attention. Sore and cracked nipples are often caused at the beginning or end of a nursing session, as a baby begins suckling improperly or as he or she is brusquely removed from the breast. When feeding your baby, be careful he or she latches on to the areola (the nipple should be in the mouth). For more preventive and healing suggestions, peruse our list below. And always check with your caregiver to make sure any creams or ointments you might use are safe for your breast-feeding baby!

- To keep your nipples from drying out, ask your caregiver to recommend a soothing cream (The Magar women of Nepal use apricot oil. The Taralpe women of Brazil apply honey.)

- Get naked. Or at least topless, especially if you're having a restful lie-down. Sore nipples are rapidly restored by contact with open air.

- If your nipple actually cracks, consult your caregiver. You may have to stop nursing from that breast for a period of time. But be sure to still pump milk in order to prevent breast engorgement.

- Treat cracked nipples by gently dabbing them with breast milk.

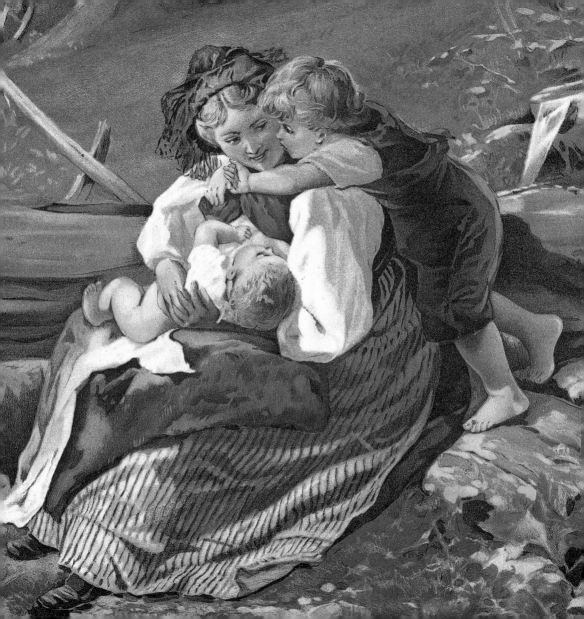

Birth is the sudden opening of a window, through which you look out upon a stupendous prospect. For what has happened? A miracle. You have exchanged nothing for the possibility of everything.

–William MacNeile Dixon

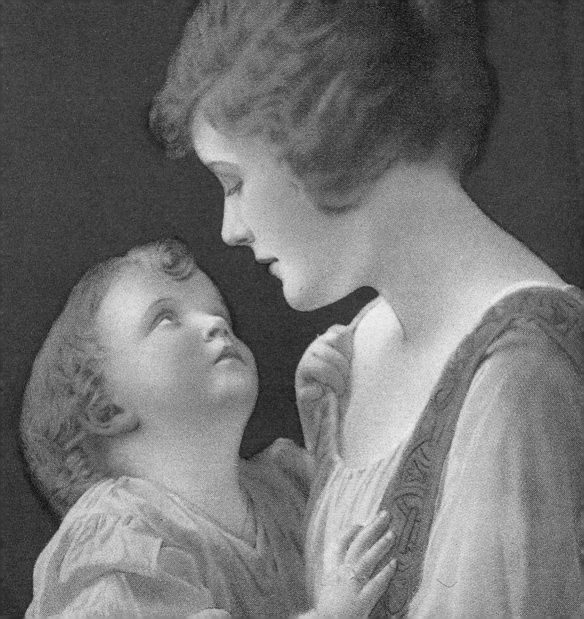

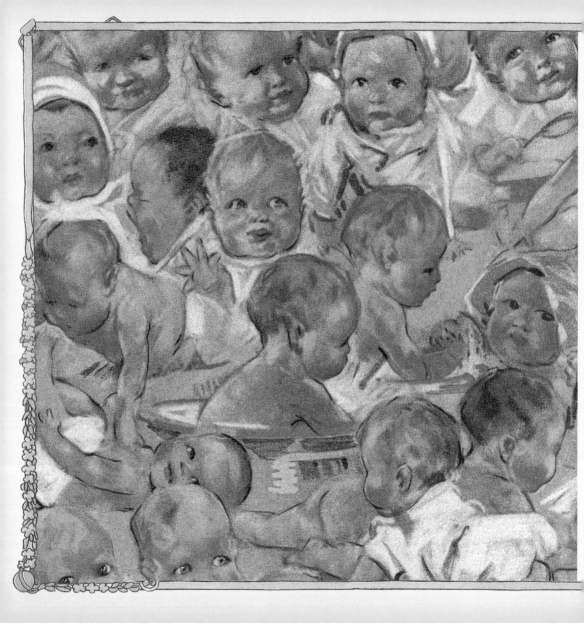

BIRTH FACTS

A baby is born every three seconds.

Between 15 and 19 sets of quintuplets are born in the U.S. every year.

The record for babies born to one woman is 69.

The lowest birth rate in the world, 1 birth per 100 people, occurs in Sweden.

About 10,501 babies are born in America daily.

Ninety-eight percent of all people alive today were born at home.

Eighty-five percent of babies are born within two weeks of their due dates.

The oldest woman to give birth was 63 years old at the time of her successful delivery in 1997.

The heaviest baby ever born weighed 29 pounds at delivery in 1939.

Sixty percent of American babies are named after close relatives.

The highest birth rate in the world, 5.3 births per 100 people, occurs in Malawi, Africa.

On the First Night

Erica Jong

On the first night
of the full moon,
the primeval sack of ocean
broke,
& I gave birth to you
little woman,
little carrot top,
little turned-up nose,
pushing you out of myself
as my mother
pushed
me out of herself,
as her mother did,
& her mother's mother
    before her,
all of us born
of woman.

I am the second daughter
of a second daughter
of a second daughter,
but you shall be the first.
You shall see the phrase
"second sex"
only in puzzlement,
wondering how anyone,
except a madman,
could call you "second"
when you are so splendidly
first,
conferring even on your
    mother
firstness, vastness, fullness
as the moon at its fullest
lights up the sky.

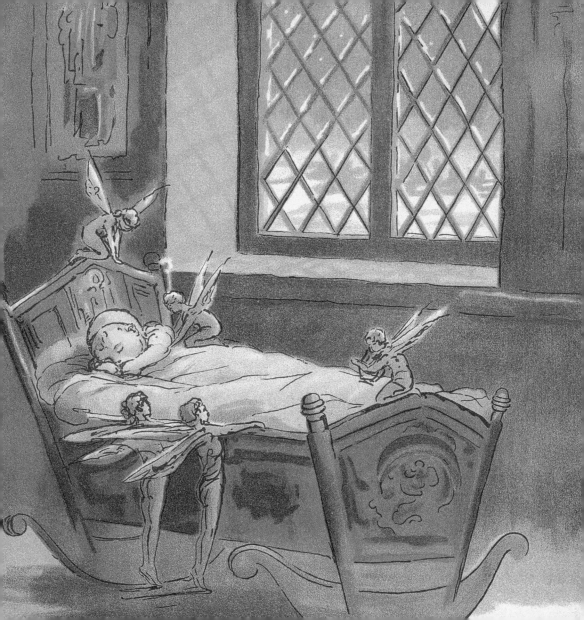

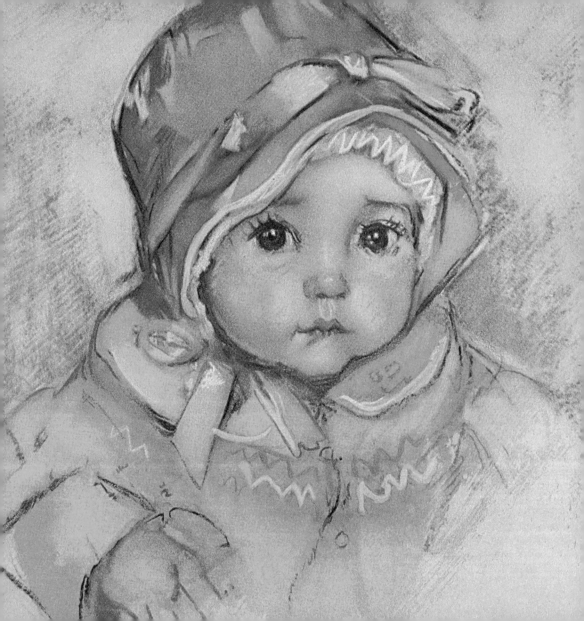

On the First Night

Now the moon is full again
& you are four weeks old.
Little lion, lioness,
yowling for my breasts,
growling at the moon,
how I love your lustiness,
your red face demanding,
your hungry mouth
    howling,
your screams, your cries
which all spell life
in large letters
the color of blood.

You are born a woman
for the sheer glory of it,
little redhead, beautiful
    screamer.

You are no second sex,
but the first of the first;
& when the moon's phases
fill out the cycle
of your life,
you will crow
for the joy
of being a woman,
telling the pallid moon
to go drown herself
in the blue ocean,
& glorying, glorying,
    glorying
in the rosy wonder
of your sunshining
    wondrous
self.

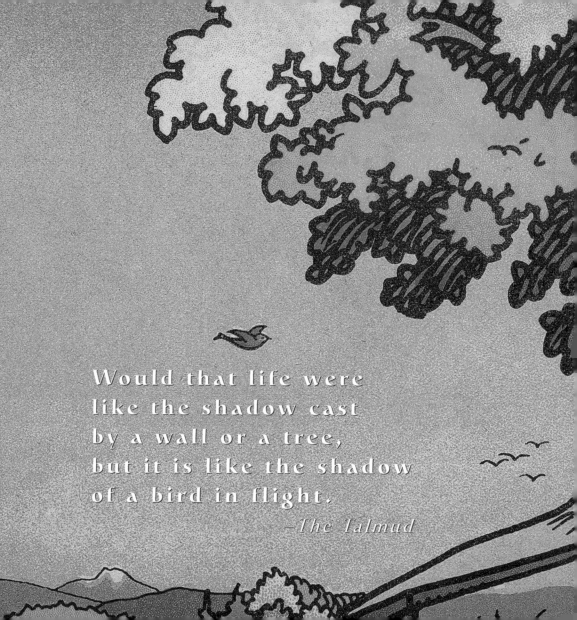

Would that life were
like the shadow cast
by a wall or a tree,
but it is like the shadow
of a bird in flight.

—*The Talmud*

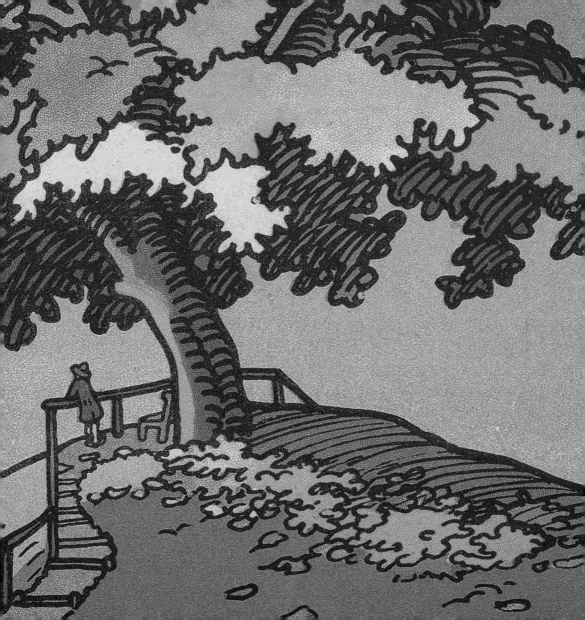

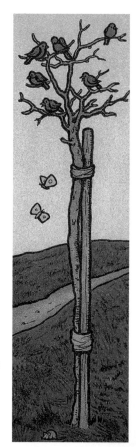

o wonder trees are often integral to birth customs. Trees symbolize the awakening of life, growth and change, our connection to nature, and our deep family roots. They provide shelter, fruits for our table, and wood for our homes. We grow trees in nurseries and cherish them, from seeds to saplings to wizened old trunks.

For the M'Benga tribe of West Africa, a tree is more than symbolic. When a child is to be born, tribe members dance round a newly planted tree believed to house the child's soul. Rich soil—best for sprouting seeds—is often likened to the mother's womb. In Australia and South Africa, want-to-be mothers literally lie in the rain so the "seeds" inside them will grow.

Trees are symbols of strength and protection. The Aztecs planted trees when their babies were born, hoping the newborns would draw strength from their vital counterparts. On the Malacca Peninsula, families plant birth trees in semi-sacred enclosures

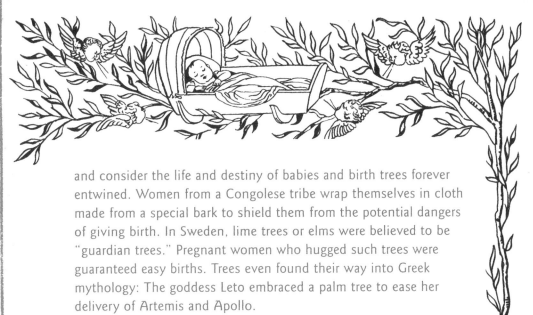

and consider the life and destiny of babies and birth trees forever
entwined. Women from a Congolese tribe wrap themselves in cloth
made from a special bark to shield them from the potential dangers
of giving birth. In Sweden, lime trees or elms were believed to be
"guardian trees." Pregnant women who hugged such trees were
guaranteed easy births. Trees even found their way into Greek
mythology: The goddess Leto embraced a palm tree to ease her
delivery of Artemis and Apollo.

Many cultures celebrate birth by planting a tree. In Haiti, a
coconut or breadfruit tree is planted to honor a newborn. The Swiss
may commemorate the birth of a girl by planting a nut or pear tree;
a boy is celebrated with an apple tree. In Ancient Palestine, Jews
planted a cedar tree, representing height and strength, when a boy
was born. A cypress tree was planted, representing tenderness and
fragrance, to honor a girl. The Jewish children were then expected to
care for their trees, and when it came time to marry, the branches
were used to make their bridal canopies.

Planting a Tree

Planting a tree is a simple, beautiful custom that gives back to nature. A child is born with an immediate companion—a living tree to care for, share birthdays with, and always return to. So create your own ritual and plant a sapling to celebrate the birth of your baby! Pick a meaningful place and a meaningful tree. Here are some suggested species and what they traditionally stand for:

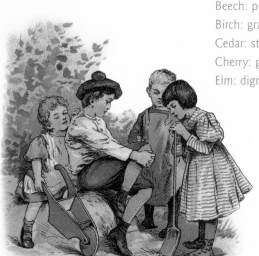

Beech: prosperity
Birch: grace
Cedar: strength
Cherry: good education
Elm: dignity

French willow: humanity
Honeysuckle: devotion
Holly: foresight
Locust: elegance
Magnolia: love of nature
Orange: generosity
Olive: peace
Pear: affection
Pine: courage
Plum: fidelity
Sycamore: curiosity
Walnut: intellect
White mulberry: wisdom
White oak: independence

How to Plant a Sapling

1. Find a location for your tree. There should have plenty of growing room both above and below the tree. Avoid pipes and other underground utilities.

2. Loosen the soil in the planting site so that it is at least twice the width of the root ball and just as deep.

3. If it's potted, remove the root ball from the pot. Otherwise, remove the twine and burlap to expose the root ball.

4. Carefully place the ball in the center of the site, such that the top of the ball is barely higher than ground level.

5. Holding the tree upright, move the displaced soil back over the ball.

6. Add water to help settle the soil and remove air pockets from around the tree.

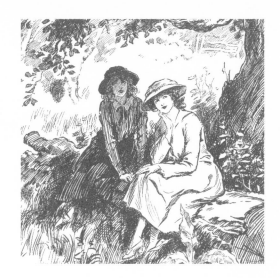

7. Only stake your sapling if you feel that it cannot stand up to the wind. Make sure that it can still flex somewhat.

8. Add 2–3 inches of bark mulch over the entire planting site, except within 6 inches of the trunk.

9. For specific planting instructions for your sapling's species, contact your local tree nursery.

Birth Announcements

It is a common Western tradition for parents to send out written cards announcing the birth of a new baby. Typically included are the date and time of birth as well as the baby's name, weight, and length, along with a photograph of the newborn.

Homemade birth announcements have a special appeal. For a personal touch, add your favorite quote about babies, birth, or having children. To craft your own announcements, use watercolor paper, which has a beautiful texture and comes in many soft colors. It's ideal for simple yet artistic cards. Cut your paper 4″ x 5″, or 10″ x 4″ for a folded card. These will fit in a standard 4 ½″ x 5 ½″ envelope. If you're looking for a unique birth announcement, here are two great suggestions.

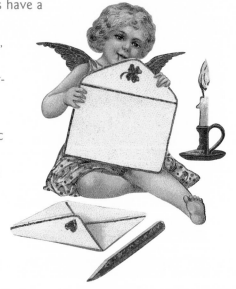

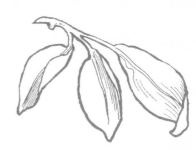

Little Diaper

1. Cut an equilateral triangle 8 inches long on each side.

2. With one point facing straight down, fold the other two points in to meet 1 inch below the middle of your inverted triangle.

3. Fold the bottom point up to the top edge, then fold the point down about an inch behind the other two points.

4. Make two small holes just below that fold and attach a large safety pin to the card.

5. Write the baby's name inside so it is visible at the top of the diaper when closed, and add the birth date, time, weight, and length below.

New Leaf Announcement

1. Cut paper 10″ x 4″ and fold in half crosswise.

2. On the front, stencil or stamp a 3- to 4-inch leaf and write your baby's name underneath.

3. On the inside, write *A new leaf on our family tree* and add the birth date, time, weight, and length. (Alternatively, you can use your computer to print this information on high-quality paper, cut to 3″ x 4″, and glue to the inside of the card.)

TRADITIONS: *Birth Announcements*

Baby is here—time to tell the world! But how? Many parents send out custom-made cards. Other moms and dads place a notice in the local paper. Farther-flung families might achieve maximum speed and coverage with an e-mailed posting and digital photographs.

But how were baby births announced before today's Internet, daily papers, and efficient postal service? The ancient Romans hung symbolic items from their front doors to announce a new birth. A piece of woolen cloth proclaimed a girl; an olive branch meant a boy.

An old Korean custom involves the parents' draping a spiraling straw rope, or *geumjul*, across their front gate to ward off evil spirits and alert visitors that a child has just been born. In one Maltese village, grateful new mothers pay the sexton to ring the church bells as thanks for their healthy infants. In Lesotho, a "surprising" old custom informs the father of the sex of the child. When a boy is born, a male neighbor sneaks up behind the father and hits him with a stick, saying, "We are given a boy!" For a girl, a woman sneaks up and douses him with a gourd full of water, saying, "The birth of a girl!"

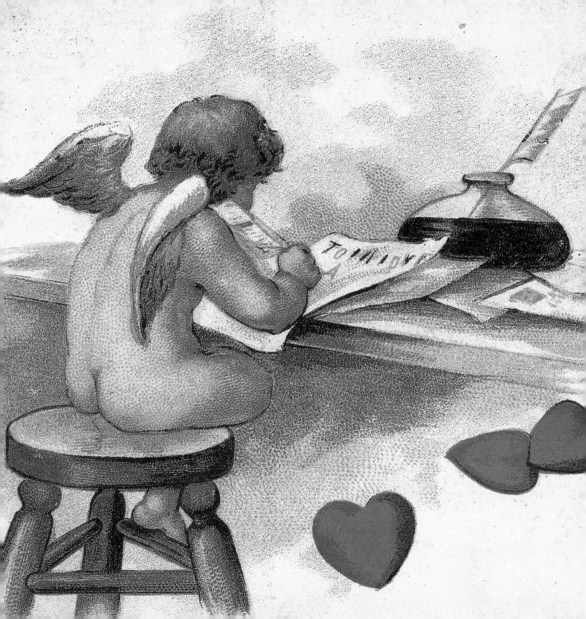

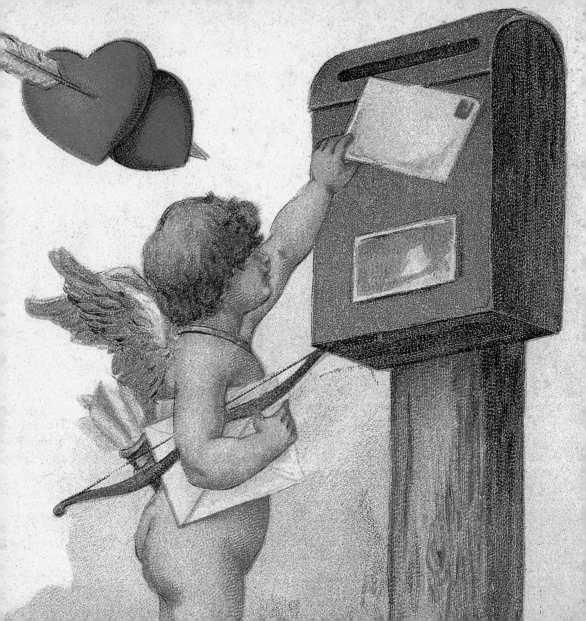

Many cultures announce and celebrate the birth of children by passing out food and gifts. The Afghani traditionally fire guns, beat drums, and give food to the poor when a baby is born, especially if it's a male child. A common Western tradition involves the father passing out cigars with pink bands for a girl; blue bands for a boy. An old tradition in the Orkney Islands has the new father bringing good luck to his child by sharing a bottle of whiskey with other local men. And in China, the father sends his in-laws money and wine, with ribbons on the bottle that specify the birth of a boy or a girl. Chinese parents also may send boxes of red eggs to family and friends when a baby is born. An odd number of eggs signifies a boy and an even number means a girl. A custom in the Netherlands is to serve *beschuit met muisjes*—sweetened biscuits with "little mice," or sugar-covered anise seeds—to all guests who come to see the new infant. Pink-and-white biscuits are for girls, and blue-and-white biscuits are for boys.

There are countless special ways to announce and celebrate your baby's birth. In one of the world's most famous birth announcements, Christians believe, the Lord sent an angel to shepherds in the fields near Bethlehem to announce the birth of the baby Jesus. Though you may not have winged messengers close at hand, take the time to find your own way to let the world know about your new little angel.

In the best of times our days are numbered. And so it would be a crime against nature for any generation to take the world's crises so solemnly that it put off enjoying those things for which we were assigned in the first place...the opportunity to do good work, to fall in love, to enjoy friends, to hit a ball and to bounce a baby.

–*Alistair Cooke*

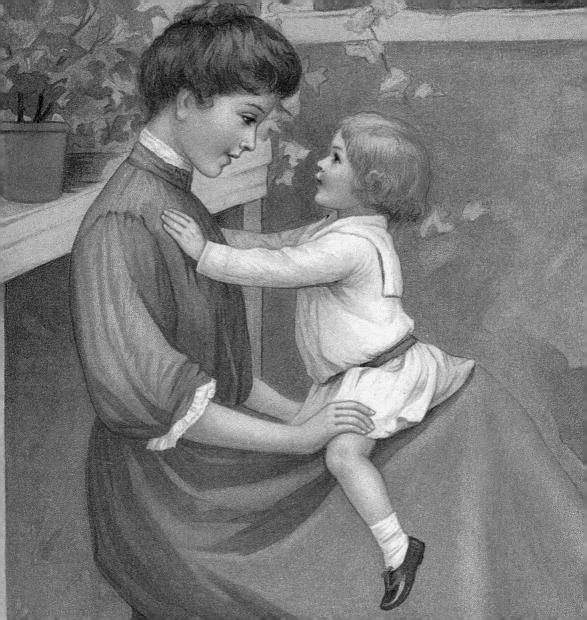

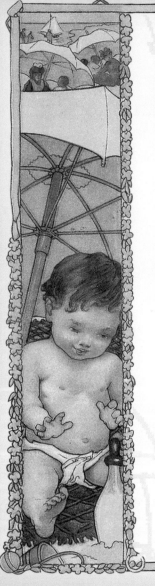

BABY FACTS

Fifteen percent of a full-term baby's body is composed of fat. Eighty percent is located beneath the skin and twenty percent around the organs.

A typical newborn doubles his weight after 6 months, and triples it in a year.

A newborn baby's head accounts for about one-fourth of her entire body weight.

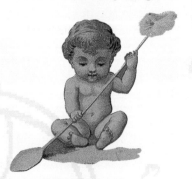

Scientists think that newborns, born with poor vision, learn to recognize their mothers by scent.

While many babies are born with blue eyes, the color may change over the next 9 months as pigment develops in the iris.

Babies can't produce tears until they are around 3–6 weeks old.

Babies are born with 300 bones, but they fuse into 206 by the time they are adults.

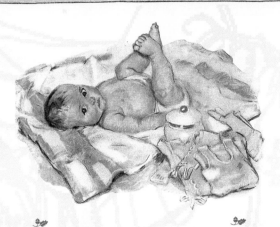

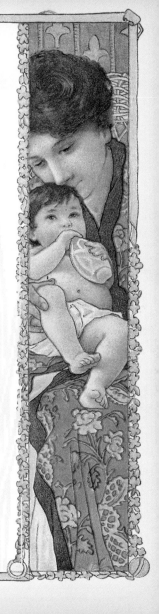

Babies born in the month of May weigh an average of 200 grams more than babies born in any other month.

Newborns have more than half a million hair follicles covering their skin.

Babies are born with fully grown fingernails and toenails, but no tear ducts.

At birth, touch is the baby's most well developed sense.

For several weeks after his birth, a baby will still assume the same fetal position it had in the womb— his muscles are used to it.

Babies are born with a "swimming reflex," and can naturally hold their breath underwater and make graceful swimming motions. They soon lose this ability, however. Some believe it may trace back to a semi-aquatic phase in recent human evolution.

How Many Children?

Surely you've thought about it. You and your partner have probably discussed it. With one on the way, it's a natural question: How many children do you plan to have? In this day and age, it's easier than ever to control the number of kids you bring into the world. But if you believe in fate, you might consider some old-fashioned methods of prediction…

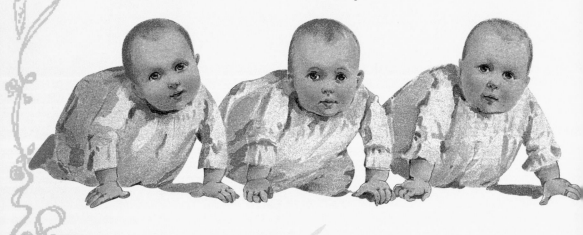

Look in the mirror and lift your eyebrows. The number of wrinkles on your forehead is said to represent your future brood. Examine your wrist. Some say the number of smaller veins stemming off from your main vein corresponds to your destined number of offspring. Form a loose fist and turn your hand to look just below your pinky finger. Between the two deepest creases you should see some smaller folds. Count the folds to see how many children you'll have. Now open your right hand. The amount of X's on your palm is yet another way to determine how big your family will grow.

For a more practiced approach, consider the ancient art of palm reading. Palm readers use the "Children Lines" to foretell your future family. To find them, look on your palm beneath your pinky finger for lines that run up and down, parallel to your fingers. The number of lines on your less-dominant hand represents how many kids you *could* have, and the lines on your dominant hand show the number of offspring you *will* have *if* you continue your life on its present course. Lighter lines represent the number of awaited girls and deeper creases correspond to boys.

At childbirth, folk wisdom holds that the number of lumps or knots on the umbilical cord of your first baby predicts how many children you will have. Also, if you cut an apple in half, the number of apple seeds showing is said to reveal the size of your future family.

And finally, an old favorite: Pick a dandelion that's gone to seed. Fill your lungs and blow. Count the number of fuzzy seeds left on the stem. See? That's how many little boys and girls you might bring into the world....

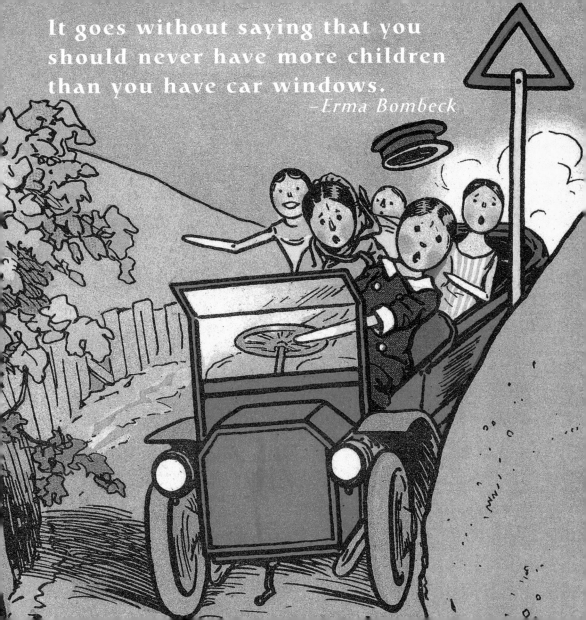

It goes without saying that you should never have more children than you have car windows.

–Erma Bombeck

The Diary of Adam

Mark Twain

Next Year

WE HAVE NAMED IT CAIN. She caught it while I was up country trapping on the North Shore of the Erie; caught it in the timber a couple of miles from our dug-out—or it might have been four, she isn't certain which. It resembles us in some ways, and may be a relation. That is what she thinks, but this is an error, in my judgment. The difference in size warrants the conclusion that it is a different and new kind of animal—a fish, perhaps, though when I put it in the water to see, it sank, and she plunged in and snatched it out before there was opportunity for the experiment to determine the matter. I still think it is a fish, but she is indifferent about what it is, and will not let me have it to try. I do not understand this. The coming of the creature seems to have changed her whole nature and made her unreasonable about experiments. She thinks more of it than she does of any of the other animals, but is not able to explain why. Her mind is disordered—everything shows it. Sometimes she carries the fish in her arms half the night when it complains and wants to get to the water. At such times the water

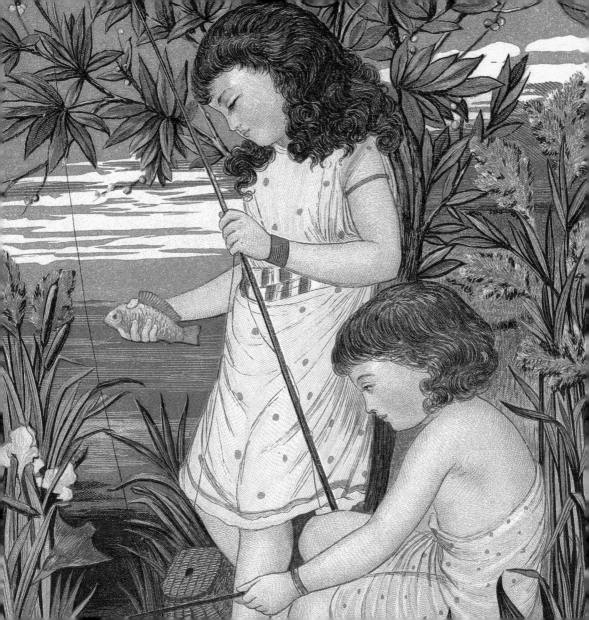

The Diary of Adam

comes out of the places in her face that she looks out of, and she pats the fish on the back and makes soft sounds with her mouth to soothe it, and betrays sorrow and solicitude in a hundred ways. I have never seen her do like this with any other fish, and it troubles me greatly. She used to carry the young tigers around so, and play with them, before we lost our property; but it was only play; she never took on about them like this when their dinner disagreed with them.

Sunday

She doesn't work Sundays, but lies around all tired out, and likes to have the fish wallow over her; and she makes fool noises to amuse it, and pretends to chew its paws, and that makes it laugh. I have not seen a fish before that could laugh. This makes me doubt.... I have come to like Sunday myself. Superintending all the week tires a body so. There ought to be more Sundays. In the old days they were tough, but now they come handy.

Wednesday

It isn't a fish. I cannot quite make out what it is. It makes curious, devilish noises when not satisfied, and says "goo-goo" when it is. It is not one of us, for it doesn't walk; it is not a bird, for it doesn't fly;

The Diary of Adam

it is not a frog, for it doesn't hop; it is not a snake, for it doesn't crawl; I feel sure it is not a fish, though I cannot get a chance to find out whether it can swim or not. It merely lies around, and mostly on its back, with its feet up. I have not seen any other animal do that before. I said I believed it was an enigma, but she only admired the word without understanding it. In my judgment it is either an enigma or some kind of a bug. If it dies, I will take it apart and see what its arrangements are. I never had a thing perplex me so.

Three Months Later

The perplexity augments instead of diminishing. I sleep but little. It has ceased from lying around, and goes about on its four legs now. Yet it differs from the other four-legged animals in that its front legs are unusually short, consequently this causes the main part of its person to stick up uncomfortably high in the air, and this is not attractive. It is built much as we are, but its method of travelling shows that it is not of our breed. The short front legs and long hind ones indicate that it is of the kangaroo family, but it is a marked variation of the species, since the true kangaroo hops, whereas this one never does. Still, it is a curious and interesting variety, and has not been catalogued before. As I discovered it, I have felt justified in securing the credit of the discovery by attaching my name to it,

The Diary of Adam

and hence have called it *Kangaroorum Adamiensis*....It must have been a young one when it came, for it has grown exceedingly since. It must be five times as big, now, as it was then, and when discontented is able to make from twenty-two to thirty-eight times the noise it made at first. Coercion does not modify this, but has the contrary effect. For this reason I discontinued the system. She reconciles it by persuasion, and by giving it things which she had previously told it she wouldn't give it. As already observed, I was not at home when it first came, and she told me she found it in the woods. It seems odd that it should be the only one, yet it must be so, for I have worn myself out these many weeks trying to find another one to add to my collection, and for this one to play with; for surely then it would be quieter, and we could tame it more easily. But I find none, nor any vestige of any; and strangest of all, no tracks. It has to live on the ground, it cannot help itself; therefore, how does it get about without leaving a track? I have set a dozen traps, but they do no good. I catch all small animals except that one; animals that merely go into the trap out of curiosity, I think, to see what the milk is there for. They never drink it.

The kangaroo still continues to grow, which is very strange and perplexing. I never knew one to be so long getting its

The Diary of Adam

growth. It has fur on its head now; not like kangaroo fur, but exactly like our hair, except that it is much finer and softer, and instead of being black is red. I am like to lose my mind over the capricious and harassing developments of this unclassifiable zoological freak. If I could catch another one— but that is hopeless; it is a new variety, and the only sample; this is plain. But I caught a true kangaroo and brought it in, thinking that this one, being lonesome, would rather have that for company than have no kin at all, or any animal it could feel a nearness to or get sympathy from in its forlorn condition here among strangers who do not know its ways or habits, or what to do to make it feel that it is among friends; but it was a mistake—it went into such fits at the sight of the kangaroo that I was convinced it had never seen one before. I pity the poor noisy little animal, but there is nothing I can do to make it happy. If I could tame it—but that is out of the question; the more I try, the worse I seem to make it. It grieves me to the heart to see it in its little storms of sorrow and passion. I wanted to let it go, but she wouldn't hear of it. That seemed cruel and not like her; and yet she may be right. It might be lonelier than ever; for since I cannot find another one, how could *it?*

The Diary of Adam

Five Months Later

It is not a kangaroo. No, for it supports itself by holding to
her finger, and thus goes a few steps on its hind legs, and
then falls down. It is probably some kind of a bear; and yet it
has no tail—as yet—and no fur, except on its head. It still
keeps on growing—that is a curious circumstance, for bears
get their growth earlier than this. Bears are dangerous—since
our catastrophe—and I shall not be satisfied to have this one
prowling about the place much longer without a muzzle on.
I have offered to get her a kangaroo if she would let this one
go, but it did no good—she is determined to run us into all
sorts of foolish risks, I think. She was not like this before she
lost her mind.

A Fortnight Later

I examined its mouth. There is no danger yet; it has only one
tooth. It has no tail yet. It makes more noise now than it ever
did before—and mainly at night. I have moved out. But I shall
go over, mornings, to breakfast, and to see if it has more teeth.
If it gets a mouthful of teeth, it will be time for it to go, tail or
no tail, for a bear does not need a tail in order to be dangerous.

The Diary of Adam

Four Months Later

I have been off hunting and fishing a month, up in the region
that she calls Buffalo; I don't know why, unless it is because
there are not any buffaloes there. Meantime the bear has
learned to paddle around all by itself on its hind legs, and says
"poppa" and "momma." It is certainly a new species. This
resemblance to words may be purely accidental, of course, and
may have no purpose or meaning; but even in that case it is still
extraordinary, and is a thing which no other bear can do. This
imitation of speech, taken together with general absence of fur
and entire absence of tail, sufficiently indicates that this is a
new kind of bear. The further study of it will be exceedingly
interesting. Meantime I will go off on a far expedition among the
forests of the North and make an exhaustive search. There must
certainly be another one somewhere, and this one will be less
dangerous when it has company of its own species. I will go
straightway; but I will muzzle this one first.

Three Months Later

It has been a weary, weary hunt, yet I have had no success. In
the mean time, without stirring from the home estate, she has

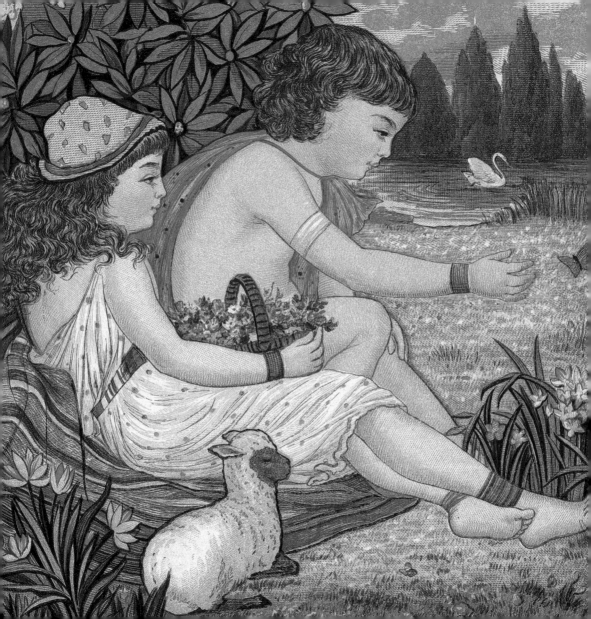

caught another one! I never saw such luck. I might have hunted these woods a hundred years, I never should have run across that thing.

Next Day

I have been comparing the new one with the old one, and it is perfectly plain that they are the same breed. I was going to stuff one of them for my collection, but she is prejudiced against it for some reason or other; so I have relinquished the idea, though I think it is a mistake. It would be an irreparable loss to science if they should get away. The old one is tamer than it was, and can laugh and talk like the parrot, having learned this, no doubt, from being with the parrot so much, and having the imitative faculty in a highly developed degree. I shall be astonished if it turns out to be a new kind of parrot; and yet I ought not to be astonished, for it has already been everything else it could think of, since those first days when it was a fish. The new one is as ugly now as the old one was at first; has the same sulphur-and-raw-meat complexion and the same singular head without any fur on it. She calls it Abel.

There Was a Child Went Forth

Walt Whitman

There was a child went forth every day,
And the first object he look'd upon, that object he became,
And that object became part of him for the day or a certain
    part of the day,
Or for many years or stretching eyeles of years.

The early lilacs became part of this child,
And grass and white and red morning-glories, and white
    and red clover, and the song of the phœbe-bird,
And the Third-month lambs and the sow's pink-faint litter,
    and the mare's foal and the cow's calf,
And the noisy brood of the barnyard or by the mire of the
    pondside,
And the fish suspending themselves so curiously below
    there, and the beautiful curious liquid,
And the water-plants with their graceful flat heads, all
    became part of him.
His own parents, he that had father'd him and she that had
    conceiv'd him in her womb and birth'd him,
They gave this child more of themselves than that,
They gave him afterward every day, they became part of him.

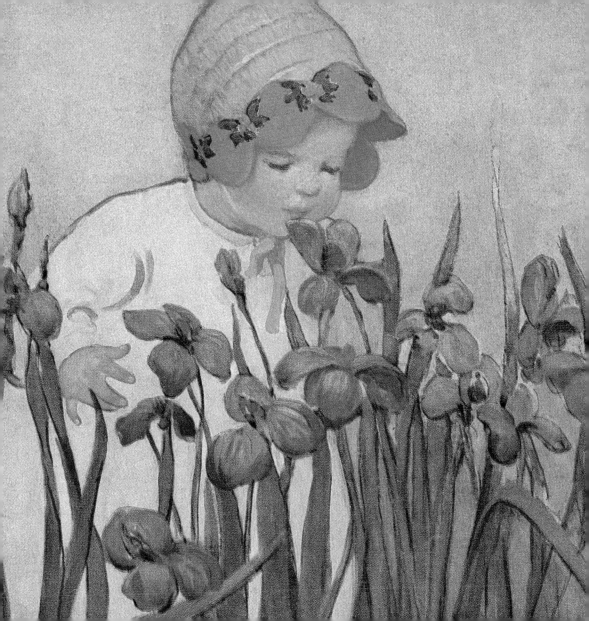

Finally, a footnote. You will never really know what kind of parent you were or if you did it right or wrong. Never. And you will worry about this and them as long as you live. But when your children have children and you watch them do what they do, you will have part of an answer.

–*Robert Fulghum*

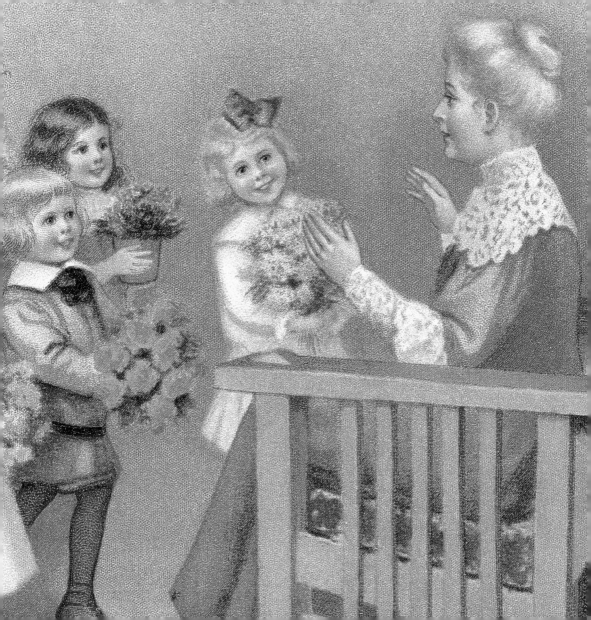

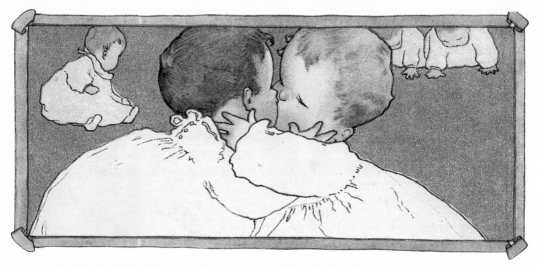

Published in 2002 by Welcome Books,
An imprint of Welcome Enterprises, Inc.
6 West 18th Street, New York, NY, 10011
(212) 989-3200; Fax (212) 989-3205
email: info@welcomebooks.biz
www.welcomebooks.biz

Designer: Jon Glick
Project Director: Katrina Fried
Editorial & Research Assistants: Lawrence Chesler,
Rachel Hertz, Nicholas Liu, Miki Raver

Home Remedies, Old Wives' Tales,
& Traditions written by Svea Vocke
Recipes by Sara Baysinger
Activities by Marsha Heckman and Sara Baysinger

Distributed to the trade in the U.S. and Canada by
Andrews McMeel Distribution Services
Order Department and Customer Service: (800) 223-2336
Orders Only Fax: (800) 943-9831

Library of Congress Control Number: 2002069999

ISBN 0-941807-72-X

Printed in Singapore
First Edition
2 4 6 8 10 9 7 5 3

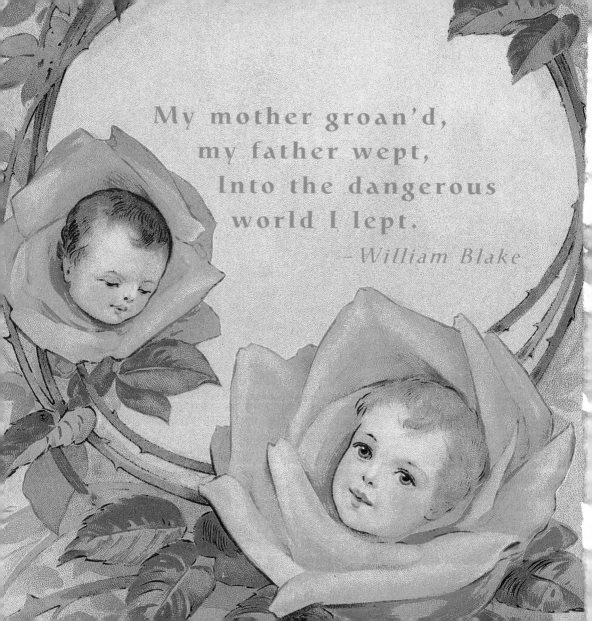

My mother groan'd,
my father wept,
Into the dangerous
world I lept.

–William Blake